Statistical Methods for Anaesthesia and Intensive Care

Commissioning editor: Melanie Tait
Editorial assistant: Myriam Brearley
Production controller: Anthony Read
Desk editor: Claire Hutchins
Cover designer: Helen Brockway

Statistical Methods for Anaesthesia and Intensive Care

Paul S Myles MB BS MPH MD FCARCSI FANZCA
Head of Research and Specialist Anaesthetist
Department of Anaesthesia and Pain Management
Alfred Hospital, Victoria
Associate Professor
Departments of Anaesthesia, and Epidemiology and Preventive
Medicine
Monash University
Melbourne, Australia

and

Tony Gin MB ChB BSc MD DipHSM FRCA FANZCA
Chairman and Chief of Service
Department of Anaesthesia and Intensive Care
Chinese University of Hong Kong
Prince of Wales Hospital
Shatin, Hong Kong

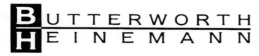

OXFORD   AUCKLAND   BOSTON   JOHANNESBURG   MELBOURNE   NEW DELHI

Butterworth-Heinemann
Linacre House, Jordan Hill, Oxford OX2 8DP
225 Wildwood Avenue, Woburn, MA 01801-2041
A division of Reed Educational and Professional Publishing Ltd

R A member of the Reed Elsevier Group

First published 2000

British Library Cataloguing in Publication Data
A catalogue record for this book is available from the British Library

Library of Congress Cataloguing in Publication Data
A catalogue record for this book is available from the Library of Congress

ISBN 0 7506 4065 0

Typeset by E & M Graphics, Midsomer Norton, Bath
Printed and bound in Great Britain by Biddles Ltd, Guildford and King's Lynn

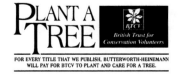

Contents

About the authors

Paul Myles is Head of Research in the Department of Anaesthesia and Pain Management at the Alfred Hospital, Melbourne. He has been a specialist anaesthetist for ten years. He received his MPH (majoring in advanced statistics and epidemiology) from Monash University in 1995 and his MD (Clinical Aspects of Cardiothoracic Anaesthesia) in 1996. He has a joint university appointment (Monash University) as Associate Professor in the Department of Anaesthesia, and Department of Epidemiology and Preventive Medicine. He is Chairman of Alfred Hospital Research Committee. He has published over 70 papers and has received more than ten peer-reviewed research grants. He is a member of three editorial boards (*Anaesthesia and Intensive Care, Asia–Pacific Heart Journal, Journal of Cardiothoracic and Vascular Anaesthesia*) and has reviewed for four others (*British Journal of Anaesthesia, Anesthesiology, Annals of Thoracic Surgery* and *Medical Journal of Australia*).

Tony Gin is Professor, Chairman and Chief of Service of the Department of Anaesthesia and Intensive Care, Chinese University of Hong Kong at the Prince of Wales Hospital, Hong Kong. He was previously Professor of the Department of Anaesthesia, Christchurch School of Medicine, University of Otago. He completed his BSc in statistics after finishing medical school and has been lecturing and examining in pharmacology and statistics in Asia and Australasia for over ten years. He has over 100 publications and has been a regular reviewer of research proposals, grant applications and manuscripts for many ethics committees, funding bodies and journals.

Paul Myles and **Tony Gin** are members of the Australian and New Zealand College of Anaesthetists' Examinations and Research Committees.

Foreword

An often puzzling, if not fearsome, aspect for an anaesthetist in training or practice, is that of grappling with 'stats'. Of course, a basic understanding of statistics is necessary in our reading of a scientific paper or in planning even the most modest research project. Books on statistics are usually written by acclaimed statisticians, they are generally helpful only to the extent that we can digest the heavy prose or the barrage of unfamiliar terms and concepts. Thankfully, *Statistical Methods for Anaesthesia and Intensive Care* will make our lives easier. The authors of this book are Tony Gin and Paul Myles, both accomplished researchers and anaesthetists. The book is written by anaesthetists for anaesthetists and clinicians, and it will lead us through the minefield of statistics that we have to cross.

Professor Teik E. Oh
President, Australian and New Zealand College of Anaesthetists
Professor, Department of Anaesthesia, University of Western Australia

Preface

'Statistics' is the science of collecting, describing and analysing data that are subject to random variation. It consists of two main areas: (i) **descriptive statistics**, whereby a collection of data is summarized in order to characterize features of its distribution, and (ii) **inferential statistics**, whereby these summary data are processed in order to estimate, or predict, characteristics of another (usually larger) group.

In most circumstances, the collection of data is from a restricted number of observations (individuals, animals or any event subject to variation); this chosen set of data is referred to as a **sample** and the reference group from which it is derived is referred to as a **population**. A population does not necessarily include all individuals, but is most often a defined group of interest, such as 'all adult surgical patients', 'all women undergoing laparoscopic surgery' or 'patients admitted to intensive care with a diagnosis of septic shock'.

So, for our purposes, statistics usually refers to the process of measuring and analysing data from a sample, in order to estimate certain characteristics of a population. These estimates of a population are most commonly an average value or proportion; and these estimates are usually compared with those of another group to determine whether one group differs significantly from the other. In order to be confident about estimation of population **parameters**, we need to be sure that our sample accurately represents our intended population. The statistical methods outlined in this book are meant to optimize this process.

Why is an understanding of statistics important for anaesthetists and intensivists? Advances in anaesthesia and intensive care rely upon development of new drugs, techniques and equipment. Evaluation and clinical application of these advances relies critically upon statistical methodology. However it is at this level that most anaesthetists and intensivists lose interest or become sceptical – this can often be attributed to the common belief that statistical analyses are misused or misrepresented. This is actually a justification for having at least a basic understanding of statistics. Accurate, reliable descriptive statistics and the correct use of inferential statistics are essential for good-quality research, and their understanding is crucial for evaluating reported advances in our specialty. In 1982, Longnecker wrote: 'If valid data are analyzed improperly, then the results become invalid and the conclusions may well be inappropriate. At best, the net effect is to waste time, effort, and money for the project. At worst, therapeutic decisions may well be based upon invalid conclusions and patients' wellbeing may be jeopardized.'*

Medical statistics is not just the use of clever mathematical formulae, but a collection of tools used to logically guide rational clinical decision-making. Our readers can be reassured that knowledge of statistics, although an essential component of the process, does not displace everyday clear thinking.

As clinicians, we want to know what management options are available for our patients, and what evidence there is to justify our choices (our patients may also want this information). How convincing is this evidence and how does it relate to our own clinical experience, or 'gut feelings'? How can we compare our own results with those of others? Under what circumstances should we change our practice? How can we show that one drug or technique is better than another, or whether a new diagnostic test adds to our clinical decision-making? Research design and statistics are tools to help clinicians make decisions. These processes are not new to medical practice, though they have recently been formalized and embraced by 'evidence-based medicine'.

Although there are many medical statistics books available on the market, in our experience they are either too mathematical in their approach or, when designed as a basic introductory textbook, use examples that have little relevance to our specialty. The design of this book is such that anaesthetists, intensivists, and trainees can systematically learn the basic principles of statistics (without boredom or frustration). This should enable the reader to successfully pass relevant examinations, design a research trial, or interpret the statistical methodology and design of a published scientific paper.

Each chapter begins with basic principles and definitions, and then explains how and why certain statistical methods are applied in clinical studies, using examples from the anaesthetic and intensive care literature. More sophisticated information is presented in brief detail, usually with reference to sources of further information for the interested reader. Note that we have highlighted **key words** in bold print. Our intention was to make it easier for readers to find specific topics within the text.

As doctors, we are expected to apply our special knowledge and training in such a way that promotes healing and good health; for anaesthetists and intensivists, this process can often be dramatic or life-saving. Progress in our specialty is rapidly evolving and acquisition of up-to-date knowledge should be based upon critical scrutiny. The aim of this book is to explain a variety of statistical principles in such a way that advances the application and development of our knowledge base, and promotes the scientific foundations of our unique specialty: anaesthesia and intensive care.

* David E. Longnecker. Support versus illumination: trends in medical statistics. Anesthesiology 1982; 57:73–74.

A cautionary tale

Three statisticians and three epidemiologists are travelling by train to a conference. The statisticians ask the epidemiologists whether they have bought tickets. They have. 'Fools!', say the statisticians, 'We've only bought one between us!' When the ticket inspector appears, the statisticians hide together in the toilet. The inspector knocks and they pass the ticket under the door. He clips the ticket and slides it back under the door to the statisticians.

The epidemiologists are very impressed, and resolve to adopt this technique themselves. On the return they purchase one ticket between them, and share the journey with the statisticians, who again ask whether they've all bought tickets. 'No', they reply, 'We've bought one to share.' 'Fools!', say the statisticians, 'We've not bought any.' 'But what will you do when the inspector comes?' 'You'll see.'

This time when the inspector appears, the epidemiologists hide together in the toilet. The statisticians walk up to the door and knock on it. The epidemiologists slide their ticket under the door, and the statisticians take it and use it as before – leaving the epidemiologists to be caught by the inspector.

The moral of this story is that you should never use a statistical technique unless you are completely familiar with it.

As retold by Frank Shann (Royal Children's Hospital, Melbourne, Australia)
The Lancet **1996; 348: 1392.**

Acknowledgements

We would like to thank Dr Rod Tayler, Dr Mark Reeves and Dr Mark Langley for their constructive criticism of earlier drafts of this book, and Dr Anna Lee for proofreading. Paul Myles would like to thank the Alfred Hospital Whole Time Medical Specialists for providing funds to purchase a notebook computer and statistical software.

We have used data from many studies, published in many journals, to illustrate some of our explanations. We would like to thank the journal publishers for permission to reproduce these results. We would particularly like to thank and acknowledge the investigators who produced the work.

Data types

Types of data
  –categorical
  –ordinal
  –numerical
Visual analogue scale (VAS)

Key points
- Categorical data are nominal and can be counted.
- Numerical data may be ordinal, discrete or continuous, and are usually measured.
- VAS measurements are ordinal data.

Types of data

Before a research study is undertaken it is important to consider the nature of the observations to be recorded. This is an essential step during the planning phase, as the type of data collected ultimately determines the way in which the study observations are described and which statistical tests will eventually be used.

At the most basic level, it is useful to distinguish between two types of data. The first type of data includes those which are defined by some characteristic, or quality, and are referred to as **qualitative data**. The second type of data includes those which are measured on a numerical scale and are referred to as **quantitative data**.

The precision with which these data are observed and recorded, and eventually analysed, is also described by a hierarchical scale (of increasing precision): **categorical**, **ordinal**, **interval** and **ratio scales** (Figure 1.1).

Categorical data

Because qualitative data are best summarized by grouping the observations into categories and counting the number in each, they are most often referred to as categorical (or nominal) data. A special case exists when there are only two categories; these are known as **dichotomous** (or binary) data.

Examples of categorical data
1. Gender
   – male
   – female

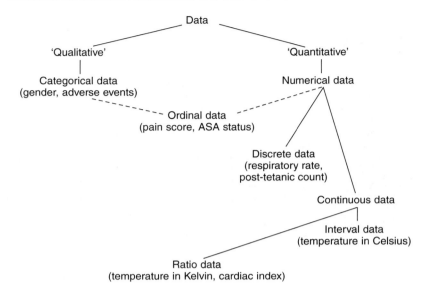

Figure 1.1 Types of data

2. Type of operation (cardiac, adult)
   – valvular
   – coronary artery
   – myocardial
   – pericardial
   – other
3. Type of ICU admission
   – medical
   – surgical
   – physical injury
   – poisoning
   – other
4. Adverse events (major cardiovascular)
   – acute myocardial infarction
   – congestive cardiac failure
   – arrhythmia
   – sudden death
   – other

The simplest way to describe categorical data is to count the number of observations in each group. These observations can then be reported using absolute count, percentages, rates or proportions.

Ordinal data

If there is a natural order among categories, so that there is a relative value among them (usually from smallest to largest), then the data can be considered as ordinal data. Although there is a semiquantitative relationship between each of the categories on an ordinal scale, there is not a direct mathematical relationship. For example, a pain score of 2 indicates more pain than a score of 1, but it does not mean twice as much pain, nor is the difference between a score of 1 and 0 equal to the difference between a score of 3 and 2.

For ordinal data, a numerical scoring system is often used to rank the categories; it may be equally appropriate to use a non-numerical record (A, B, C, D; or +, ++, +++, ++++). A numerical scoring system does, however, have practical usage, particularly for the convenience of data recording and eventual statistical analyses. Nevertheless, ordinal data are, strictly speaking, a type of categorical data. Once again these observations can be described by an absolute count, percentages, rates or proportions. Ordinal data can also be summarized by the median value and range (see Chapter 2).

Examples of ordinal data
1. Pain score
   0 = no pain
   1 = mild pain
   2 = moderate pain
   3 = severe pain
   4 = unbearable pain
2. Extent of epidural block:
   A = lumbar (L1–L5)
   B = low thoracic (T10–T12)
   C = mid-thoracic (T5–T9)
   D = high thoracic (T1–T4)
3. Preoperative risk:
   ASA* I/II = low risk
   ASA III = mild risk
   ASA IV = moderate risk
   ASA V = high risk

Numerical data

Quantitative data are more commonly referred to as numerical data; these observations can be subdivided into discrete and continuous measurements. Discrete numerical data can only be recorded as whole numbers (integers), whereas continuous data can assume any value. Put simply, observations that are counted are discrete numerical data and observations that are measured are usually continuous data.

Examples of numerical data
1. Episodes of myocardial ischaemia (discrete)
2. Body weight (continuous)
3. Creatinine clearance (continuous)
4. Cardiac index (continuous)

---

* ASA = American Society of Anesthesiologists' physical status classification.

5. Respiratory rate (discrete/continuous)
6. Post-tetanic count (discrete)

There are circumstances where data are recorded on a **discrete scale**, but may be considered as continuous data, if it is conceptually possible to achieve any value throughout the possible range of values (even if the observations are not recorded as such, or eventual statistical analysis does not consider this possible precision). For example, although respiratory rate is generally considered to only have discrete values, and is usually recorded as such, it is possible that any value may exist (at any one time) and a value of, say, 9.4 breaths/min is meaningful. This would not be the case, for example, with number of episodes of myocardial ischaemia.

It has to be admitted that the distinction between discrete and continuous numerical data is sometimes blurred, so that discrete data may assume the properties of continuous data if there is a large range of potential values.

Continuous data can also be further subdivided into either an **interval** or **ratio scale**, whereby data on a ratio scale have a true zero point and any two values can be numerically related, resulting in a true ratio. The classic example of this is the measurement of temperature. If temperatures are measured on a Celsius scale they are considered interval data, but when measured on a Kelvin scale they are ratio data: 0°C is not zero heat, nor is 26°C twice as hot as 13°C. However, this distinction has no practical significance for our purposes, as both types of continuous data are recorded and reported in the same way, and are dealt with using the same statistical methods.

Numerical data are usually reported as mean and standard deviation, or as median and range (see Chapter 2).

In general, the observations of interest in a research study are also referred to as variables, in that they can have different values (i.e. they can vary). So that, for example, gender may be referred to as a categorical or dichotomous variable, and cardiac index as a continuous variable. Studies may include more than one type of data.

For example, in a study investigating the comparative benefits of patient controlled analgesia after cardiac surgery, Myles et al.[1] recorded the following outcomes: pain score, where 0 = no pain, 1 = mild pain, 2 = moderate pain, 3 = severe pain and 4 = unbearable pain (these are ordinal data); incidence of respiratory depression (categorical data); total morphine consumption (continuous data) and serum cortisol level (continuous data).

As another example, Gutierrez et al.[2] investigated whether outcome in the ICU could be improved with therapy guided by measurement of gastric intramucosal pH (pHi). Outcomes of interest included number of organs failed in each patient (discrete data), incidence of organ failure (categorical data), pHi (continuous data) and blood pressure (continuous data). They also recorded therapeutic interventions, including the therapeutic intervention scoring system (TISS) (ordinal data), use of inotrope infusions (categorical data) and bicarbonate administration (yes/no: dichotomous, categorical data).

Visual analogue scale (VAS)

A frequently used tool in anaesthesia research is the 100 mm visual analogue scale (VAS).[3] This is most commonly used to measure postoperative pain, but can also be used to measure a diverse range of (mostly) subjective experiences such as preoperative anxiety, postoperative nausea, and patient satisfaction after ICU discharge. Because there are infinite possible values that can occur throughout the range 0–100 mm, describing a continuum of pain intensity, most researchers treat the resulting data as continuous.[4,5] If there is some doubt about the sample distribution, then the data should be considered ordinal.

There has been some controversy in the literature regarding which statistical tests should be used when analysing VAS data.[4,5] Some statistical tests (**'parametric tests'**) assume that sample data have been taken from a normally distributed population. Mantha *et al.*[4] surveyed the anaesthetic literature and found that approximately 50% used parametric tests. Dexter and Chestnut[5] used a multiple resampling (of VAS data) method to demonstrate that parametric tests had the greater **power** to detect differences among groups.

Myles *et al.*[6] have recently shown that the VAS has properties consistent with a linear scale, and thus VAS scores can be treated as ratio data. This supports the notion that a change in the VAS score represents a relative change in the magnitude of pain sensation. This enhances its clinical application.

Nevertheless, when small numbers of observations are being analysed (say, less than 30 observations), it is preferable to consider VAS data as ordinal.

For a number of practical reasons, a VAS is sometimes converted to a **'verbal rating scale'**, whereby the subject is asked to rate an endpoint on a scale of 0–10 (or 0–5), most commonly recorded as whole numbers. In this situation it is preferable to treat the observations as ordinal data.

Changing data scales
Although data are characterized by the nature of the observations, the precision of the recorded data may be reduced so that continuous data become ordinal, or ordinal data become categorical (even dichotomous). This may occur because the researcher is not confident with the accuracy of their measuring instrument, is unconcerned about loss of fine detail, or where group numbers are not large enough to adequately represent a variable of interest. In most cases, however, it simply makes clinical interpretation easier and this is the most valid and prevalent in the medical literature.

For example, smoking status can be recorded as smoker/non-smoker (categorical data), heavy smoker/light smoker/ex-smoker/non-smoker (ordinal data), or by the number of cigarettes smoked per day (discrete data).

Another example is the detection of myocardial ischaemia using ECG ST-segment monitoring – these are actually continuous numerical data, whereby the extent of ST-segment depression is considered to represent the degree of myocardial ischaemia. For several reasons, it is generally accepted that ST-segment depression greater than 1.0 mm indicates myocardial ischaemia, so that ST-segment depression less than this value is categorized as 'no ischaemia' and that beyond 1.0 mm as 'ischaemia'. [7] This results in a loss of detail, but has widespread clinical acceptance (see Chapter 8 for further discussion of this issue).

References

1. Myles PS, Buckland MR, Cannon GB *et al.* Comparison of patient-controlled analgesia and nurse-controlled infusion analgesia after cardiac surgery. *Anaesth Intensive Care* 1994; **22**:672–678.
2. Gutierrez G, Palizas F, Doglio G *et al.* Gastric mucosal pH as a therapeutic index of tissue oxygenation in critically ill patients. *Lancet* 1992; **339**:195–199.
3. Revill SI, Robinson JO, Rosen M *et al.* The reliability of a linear analogue for evaluating pain. *Anaesthesia* 1976; **31**:1191–1198.
4. Mantha S, Thisted R, Foss J *et al.* A proposal to use confidence intervals for visual analog scale data for pain measurement to determine clinical significance. *Anesth Analg* 1993; **77**:1041–1047.
5. Dexter F, Chestnut DH. Analysis of statistical tests to compare visual analogue scale data measurements among groups. *Anesthesiology* 1995; **82**:896–902.
6. Myles PS, Troedel S, Boquest M, Reeves M. The pain visual analogue scale: is it linear or non-linear? *Anesth Analg* 1999; **89**:1517–1520.
7. Fleisher L, Rosenbaum S, Nelson A *et al.* The predictive value of preoperative silent ischemia for postoperative ischemic cardiac events in vascular and nonvascular surgical patients. *Am Heart J* 1991; **122**:980–986.

2

Descriptive statistics

Measures of central tendency	Confidence intervals
–mode	Frequency distributions
–median	–normal
–mean	–binomial
Degree of dispersion	–Poisson
–range	**Data transformation**
–percentiles	**Rates and proportions**
–variance	**Incidence and prevalence**
–standard deviation	**Presentation of data**
–standard error	

Key points
- The central tendency of a frequency distribution can be described by the mean, median or mode.
- The mean is the average value, median the middle value, and mode the most common value.
- Degree of dispersion can be described by the range of values, percentiles, standard deviation or variance.
- Standard error is a measure of precision and can be used to calculate a confidence interval.
- Most biological variation has a normal distribution, whereby approximately 95% of observations lie within two standard deviations of the mean.
- Data transformation can be used to produce a more normal distribution.

Descriptive statistics summarize a collection of data from a sample or population. Traditionally summaries of sample data ('**statistics**') are defined by Roman letters ($\bar{x}$, s_x, etc.) and summaries of population data ('**parameters**') are defined by Greek letters (μ, σ, etc.).

Individual observations within a sample or population tend to cluster about a central location, with more extreme observations being less frequent. The extent that observations cluster can be described by the **central tendency**. The spread can be described by the **degree of dispersion**.

For example, if 13 anaesthetic registrars have their cardiac output measured at rest, their results may be: 6.2, 4.9, 4.7, 5.9, 5.2, 6.6, 5.0, 6.1, 5.8, 5.6, 7.0, 6.6 and 5.5 l/min. How can their data be summarized in order to best represent the observations, so that we can compare their cardiac output data with other groups?

The most simple approach is to **rank** the observations, from lowest to highest: 4.7, 4.9, 5.0, 5.2, 5.5, 5.6, 5.8, 5.9, 6.1, 6.2, 6.6, 6.6 and 7.0 l/min. We now have a clearer idea of what the typical cardiac output might be, because we can identify a middle value or a commonly occurring value (the smallest or largest value is least likely to represent our sample group).

Measures of central tendency

The sample **mode** is the most common value. In the example above it is 6.6 l/min. This may not be the best method of summarizing the data (in our example it occurs twice, not much more frequent than other observations).

If the sample is ranked, the **median** is the middle value. If there is an even number of observations, then the median is calculated as the average of the two middle values. In the example above it is 5.8 l/min.

The **mean** (or more correctly, the **arithmetic mean**) is the average value. It is calculated as the sum of (depicted by the Greek letter, Σ) the observations, divided by the number of observations. The formula for the mean is:

$$\text{mean, } \bar{x} = \frac{\Sigma x}{n}$$

where x = each observation, and n = number of observations. In the example, the mean can be calculated as $75.1/13 = 5.78$ l/min.

The mean is the most commonly used single measure to summarize a set of observations. It is usually a reliable measure of central tendency.

Degree of dispersion

The spread, or variability, of a sample can be readily described by the minimum and maximum values. The difference between them is the **range**. In the example above, the range is $(7.0 - 4.7)$ 2.3 l/min. The range does not provide much information about the overall distribution of observations, and is also heavily affected by extreme values.

A clearer description of the observations can be obtained by ranking the data and grouping them into **percentiles**. Percentiles rank observations into 100 equal parts. We then have more information about the pattern of spread. We can describe 25%, 50%, 75%, or any other amount of observations. The median is the 50th centile. If we include the middle 50% of the observations about the median (25th to 75th centile), we have the **interquartile range**. In the example above, the interquartile range is 5.2–6.1 l/min.

A better method of measuring variability about the mean is to see how closely each individual observation clusters about it. The **variance** is such a method. It sums the square of each difference ('**sum of squares**') and divides by the number of observations. The formula for variance is:

$$s_x^2 = \frac{\Sigma(x - \bar{x})^2}{n - 1}$$

The expression within the parentheses is squared so that it removes negative values. The formula for the variance (and standard deviation, see below) for a population has the value 'n' as the denominator. The expression '$n - 1$' is known as the **degrees of freedom** and is one less than the number of observations. This is explained by a defined number of observations in a sample with a known mean – each observation is free to vary except the last one which must be a defined value.

The degrees of freedom describe the number of independent observations or choices available. Consider a situation where four numbers must add up to ten and one can choose the four numbers (n = 4). Provided that one does not choose the largest remainder, it is possible to have free choice in choosing the first three numbers, but the last number is fixed by the first three choices. The degee of freedom was $(n - 1)$.

The degrees of freedom is used when calculating the variance (and standard deviation) of a sample because the sample mean is a predetermined estimate of the population mean (each individual in the sample is a random selection, but not the fixed sample mean value).

The variance is measured in units of x^2. This is sometimes difficult to comprehend and so we often use the square root of variance in order to retain the basic unit of observation. The positive square root of the variance is the **standard deviation** (SD or s_x).

The formula for SD is:

$$s_x = \sqrt{\left(\frac{\Sigma(x - \bar{x})^2}{n - 1}\right)}$$

In the example above, SD can be calculated as 0.714 l/min.

Another measure of variability is the **coefficient of variation** (CV). This considers the relative size of the SD with respect to the mean. It is commonly used to describe variability of measurement instruments. It is generally accepted that a CV of less than 5% is acceptable reproducibility.

CV = SD/mean × 100%

There are many sources of variability in data collection. Biological variability – variation between individuals and over time – is a fundamental source of scatter. Another source of variability is measurement imprecision (this can be quantified by the CV). These types of variability result in **random error**. Lastly, there are mistakes or biases in measurement or recording. This is **systematic error**. Determined efforts should be made to minimize random and systematic error. Random error can be reduced by use of accurate measurement instruments, taking multiple measurements, and using trained observers. The ability to detect differences between groups is blurred by large variance, and this inflates the sample size that is needed to be studied. Systematic error cannot be compensated for by increasing sample size.

Another measure of variability is the **standard error** (SE). It is calculated from the SD and sample size (n):

$$SE = \frac{SD}{\sqrt{n}}$$

Standard error is a much smaller numerical value than SD and is often presented (wrongly) for this reason. It is not meant to be used to describe variability of sample data.[1–5] It is used to estimate a population parameter from a sample – it is a measure of precision.

Standard error is also known as the standard error of the mean. If one takes a number of samples from a population, we will have a mean for each sample. The SD of the sample means is the standard error.

In the example above we selected 13 individuals and measured their cardiac outputs. If we now selected a second group of (say) 11 individuals ($n = 11$), and then a third ($n = 8$), a fourth ($n = 13$), and perhaps a fifth ($n = 15$), we would have five different sample means. Each may have sampled from the same population (in our example these may be anaesthetic registrars within a regional training programme) and so each sample could be used to estimate the true population mean and the SD. The five sample means would have their own distribution and it would be expected to have less dispersion than that of all the individuals in the samples, i.e.

sample A ($n = 13$) mean 5.78 l/min
sample B ($n = 11$) mean 5.54 l/min
sample C ($n = 8$) mean 5.99 l/min
sample D ($n = 13$) mean 6.12 l/min
sample E ($n = 15$) mean 5.75 l/min
mean (of 5 samples): 5.84 l/min
SD of the 5 sample means: 0.23 l/min

The SE represents the SD of the sample means (0.23 l/min). But we do not generally take multiple samples and are left to determine the SE from one sample. The example above (sample A) has an SD of 0.714 and an SE of (0.714/3.61) = 0.20 l/min.

In general we are not interested in the characteristics of multiple samples, but more specifically how reliable our one sample is in describing the true population. We use SE to define a range in which the true population mean value should lie.

Standard error is used to calculate **confidence intervals**, and so is a measure of precision (of how well sample data can be used to predict a population parameter). If the sample is very large (with a large value of n), then prediction becomes more reliable. Large samples increase precision. We stated above that random error can be compensated for by increasing sample size. This is an inefficient (and possibly costly) method, as a halving of SE requires a four-fold increase in sample size ($\sqrt{4} = 2$).

Confidence intervals

Confidence intervals are derived from the SE and define a range of values that are likely to include a population parameter. The two ends of the range are called **confidence limits**.

The width of the confidence interval depends on the SE (and thus sample size, n) and the degree of confidence required (say 90, 95 or 99%) : 95% confidence intervals (95% CI) are most commonly used. The range, 1.96 standard errors either side of the sample mean, has a 95% probability of including the population mean; and 2.58 standard errors either side of the sample mean has a 99% probability of including the population mean, i.e.

95% CI of the mean = sample mean ± (1.96 × SE)

The 95% CI should be distinguished from a property of the normal distribution where 95% of observations lie within 1.96 standard deviations of the mean. The 95% CI relates to the sample statistic (e.g. mean), *not* the individual observations. In a similar way, the SD indicates the spread of individual observations in the sample, while the SE of the mean relates the sample mean to the true population mean.

In our example above, 95% CI can be calculated as the mean (5.78) ± (1.96 × 0.198), that is 5.39 to 6.17 l/min. This states that the probability (*P*) of the true population cardiac output lying within this range is *P* = 0.95, or 95%. It can also be stated that 95% of further sample means would lie in this range.

Confidence intervals can be used to estimate most population parameters from sample statistics (means, proportions, correlation coefficients, regression coefficients, risk ratios, etc. – see later chapters). They are all calculated from SE (but each has a different formula to estimate its SE).

Example 2.1 A set of observations: creatinine clearance values (*x*, ml/min) in 15 critically ill patients. IQR = interquartile range, CI = confidence interval

Patient	x	$x - \bar{x}$	$(x - \bar{x})^2$	
1	76	8.54	72.9	
2	100	32.54	1059	
3	46	−21.46	4620	
4	65	−2.46	6.1	range = 81 (26 to 107)
5	89	11.54	133	mode = 76
6	37	−30.46	928	median = 68
7	59	−8.46	71.6	IQR = 52.5 to 82.5
8	68	0.54	0.25	
9	107	39.54	1563	
10	26	−41.46	1719	
11	38	−29.46	868	
12	90	22.54	508	
13	75	7.54	56.9	
14	76	8.54	72.9	
15	60	−7.46	55.7	
total (Σ) = 1012			7930	

mean, $\bar{x}$ = 1012/15 = 67.46
SD = √(7930/14) = 23.8
SE = 23.8/3.87 = 6.14
95% CI of the mean = 55.4 to 79.5

Frequency distributions

It is useful to summarize a number of observations with a **frequency distribution**. This is a set of all observations and their frequencies. They may be summarized in a table or a graph (see also Figures 2.1 and 2.2).

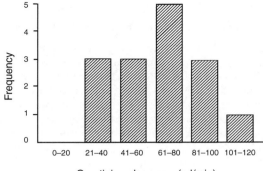

Figure 2.1 A bar diagram of the distribution of creatinine clearance values in critically ill patients

Example 2.2 From Example 2.1 we can summarize the frequency distribution of creatinine clearance values (CrCl, ml/min) when categorized into intervals

CrCl interval	Frequency	Relative frequency	Cumulative frequency
0–20	0	0	0
21–40	3	0.2	0.20
41–60	3	0.2	0.40
61–80	5	0.33	0.73
81–100	3	0.2	0.93
101–120	1	0.07	1.0

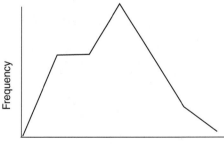

Creatinine clearance (ml/min)

Figure 2.2 A frequency distribution curve of creatinine clearance values in critically ill patients

Normal distribution

Most biological variation has a tendency to cluster around a central value, with a symmetrical positive and negative deviation about this point, and more extreme values becoming less frequent the further they lie from the central point. These features describe a **normal distribution** and can be plotted as a normal distribution curve. It is sometimes referred to as a Gaussian distribution after the German mathematician, Gauss (1777–1855).

If we now look at the formula for the normal distribution, we can see that there are two parameters that define the curve, namely μ (mu, the mean) and σ (sigma, the standard deviation); the other terms are constants:

$$f(x) = \frac{1}{\sigma\sqrt{2\pi}}\, e^{-1/2(x-\mu)^2/\sigma^2}$$

The standard normal distribution curve (Figure 2.3) is a symmetrical bell-shaped curve with a mean of 0 and a standard deviation of 1. This is also known as the **z distribution**. It can be defined by the following equation:

$$f(x) = \frac{1}{\sqrt{2\pi}}\, e^{(-1/2 x^2)}$$

A **z transformation** converts any normal distribution curve to a standard normal distribution curve, with mean = 0, SD = 1. The formula for z is:

$$z = \frac{x - \mu}{\text{SD}}$$

where μ = mean. This results in a **standardized score**, *z*, i.e. the number of standard deviations from the mean in a standard normal distribution curve. It can be used to determine probability (by referring to a *z* table in a reference book).

Using Example 2.1 above, we can determine the probability of a creatinine clearance value less than 40 ml/min if we assume that the sample data are derived from a normal distribution and the sample mean and SD represent that population:

$$z = \frac{40 - 67.5}{23.8} = 1.16$$

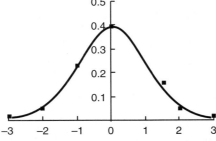

Figure 2.3 The standard normal distribution curve (mean 0, standard deviation 1.0)

If we refer to a z table in a reference book we will find that a z value of 1.16 corresponds to a (one-tailed) P value of 0.12. This means that the probability of a critically ill patient having a creatinine clearance of less than 40 ml/min is 0.12 (or 12%). In other words, it would not be considered a very uncommon event in this population.

As the number of observations increases (say, $n > 100$), the shape of a sampling distribution will approximate a normal distribution curve even if the distribution of the variable in question is not normal. This is explained by the **central limit theorem**, and indicates why the normal distribution is so important in medical research.

The normal distribution curve has a central tendency and a degree of dispersion. The mode, median and mean of this curve are the same. The probability is equal to the area under the curve. In a normal distribution, one SD either side of the mean includes 68% of the total area, two standard deviations 95.4%, and three standard deviations 99.7%. 95% of the population lie within 1.96 standard deviations.

Many statistical techniques have assumptions of normality of the data. It is not necessary for the sample data to be normally distributed, but it should represent a population that is normally distributed.[5,6] It is preferable to be able to demonstrate this, either graphically or by using a **'goodness of fit'** test (see Chapters 5 and 11).

In some circumstances there is an asymmetric distribution (**skew**), so that one of the tails is elongated. If a distribution is skewed, then the measures of central tendency will differ. If the distribution is skewed to the right, then the median will be smaller than the mean. The median is a better measure of central tendency in a skewed distribution. If sample data are skewed, they can first be transformed into a normal distribution, and then analysed (see below). **Kurtosis** describes how peaked the distribution is. The kurtosis of a normal distribution is zero.

A **bimodal distribution** consists of two peaks and suggests that the sample is not homogeneous but possibly represents two different populations.

Binomial distribution

A **binomial distribution** exists if a population contains items which belong to one of two mutually exclusive categories (A or B), e.g.

male/female
complication/no complication

It has the following conditions:

1. There are a fixed number of observations (trials)
2. Only two outcomes are possible
3. The trials are independent
4. There is a constant probability for the occurrence of each event

The binomial distribution describes the probability of events in a fixed number of observations, i.e.

if $P(A) = \pi$, then $P(B) = 1 - \pi$

if no. of observations $= n$ and number of A $= r$, then number of B $= n - r$

The probability of any event in a binomial distribution can be calculated from this formula:

$$P(r) = \binom{n}{r} \pi^r (1 - \pi)^{n-r}$$

Example 2.3 If previous experience suggests that 20% of patients require overnight admission to hospital after laparoscopic surgery, what will be the likelihood of exactly two patients being admitted after a list of nine cases?

i.e. $\pi = 0.20$, $n = 9$, $r = 2$

$$P(2) = \binom{9}{2} 0.2^2 (1 - 0.2)^7$$

$$P(2) = \frac{9.8}{2.1} 0.2^2 (1 - 0.2)^7 = 36.(0.04).(0.21) = 0.30$$

In this example, the probability of two patients being admitted is approximately 30%.

If the number of observations is very large, and the probability of an event is small, then calculation of binomial probabilities can be quite tedious. An approximation known as the **Poisson distribution** can be used.

Poisson distribution

A Poisson distribution is calculated from an exponential formula, and calculates the probability of events in a fixed time interval. It is used to describe rare, random processes. It has a single parameter, λ, which is both the mean and the variance:

$$P(r) = \frac{\lambda^r}{r!} e^{-\lambda}$$

The Poisson distribution has the following conditions:

1. Events occur randomly
2. Events occur independently
3. Events occur uniformly and singly

Example 2.4 If there were 122 late (after 8 pm) admissions to a post-anaesthetic recovery room over a one-year period (thus mean rate, $\lambda = 0.33$/day), what is the probability of (say) more than one late admission occurring on any one day? (This query may have relevance if planning staffing levels)

$\lambda = 0.33$	$r > 1$
$P(0) = e^{-0.33} = 0.72$	and $P(1) = e^{-0.33}(1 + 0.33) = 0.24$
thus, $P(0 \text{ or } 1) = 0.96$	and so $P(> 1) = 0.04$

Thus, the probability that more than one patient would be admitted after 8 pm is 4%.

Data transformation

In some circumstances it may be preferable to transform a distribution so that it approximates a normal distribution. This generally equalizes group variances, and makes data analyses and interpretation easier.[6] This is a useful approach if sample data are skewed.

The most commonly used transformation is a **log transformation**. This can result in a mean that is independent of the variance, a characteristic of a normal distribution.[6]

The antilog of the mean of a set of logarithms is a **geometric mean**. It is a good measure of central tendency if a distribution is skewed.

Rates and proportions

A **rate** is a measure of the frequency of an event. It consists of a numerator (number of events) and a denominator (number in the population). For example, if 14 colorectal surgical patients have died in a hospital performing 188 cases in the previous 12 months, the reported mortality rate would be 14/174 (= 0.0805), or 8.05%. Note that a rate does not include the number of events in the denominator.

A **proportion** includes the numerator within the denominator. It has a value between 0 and 1.0, and can be multiplied by 100% to give a **percentage**. In our colorectal surgical example, the proportion of deaths is 14/188 (= 0.0745), or 7.45%. Rates are sometimes used interchangeably with proportions (e.g. mortality 'rates' often include the deaths in the denominator). This is a common practice that is generally accepted.

Two proportions may be compared by combining them as a **ratio**. For example, a **risk ratio** is the incidence rate of an event in an exposed population versus the incidence rate in a non-exposed population. If the risk ratio is greater than 1.0, there is an increased risk with that exposure.

Incidence and prevalence

Incidence and prevalence are often used interchangeably, but they are different and this difference should be understood. **Incidence** is the number of individuals who develop a disease (i.e. new case) in a given time period. The incidence rate is an estimate of the probability, or risk, of developing a disease in a specified time period.

Prevalence is the current number of cases (pre-existing and new). Prevalence is a proportion, obtained by dividing the number of individuals with the disease by the number of people in the population.

Presentation of data

The mean is the most commonly used single measure to summarize a set of observations. It is usually a reliable measure of central tendency. This is because most biological variation is symmetrically distributed about a central location. Mean and SD are the best statistics to use when describing data from a normal distribution.

It has been suggested that the correct method for presentation of normally distributed sample data variability is mean (SD) and not mean (± SD).[7] The '±' symbol implies that we are interested in the range of one SD above and below the mean; we are generally more interested in the degree of spread of the sample data.

One of the weaknesses of the mean is that it is affected by extreme values. In these circumstances it may be preferable to use median or geometric mean as a measure of central tendency, and range or inter-quartile range for degree of spread. The mode is best used if the data have a bimodal distribution.

Ordinal data should be described with mode or median, or each category as number (%). Categorical data can be presented as number (%).

A **box and whisker plot** (Figure 2.4) can be used to depict median, interquartile range and range. For example, we can use our data from Example 2.1 and depict the median (line through box), interquartile range (box) and whiskers (5% and 95% centiles, or minimum and maximum).

Tables and diagrams are convenient ways of summarizing data. They should be clearly labelled and self-explanatory, and as simple as possible. Most journals include specific guidelines and these should be followed.

Tables should have their rows and columns labelled. Excessive detail or numerical precision (say, beyond 3 significant figures) should be avoided. Graph axes and scales should be labelled. If the axis does not begin at the origin (zero), then a break in the axis should be included.

On some occasions it may be acceptable to use standard error bars on graphs (for ease of presentation), but on these occasions they should be clearly labelled.

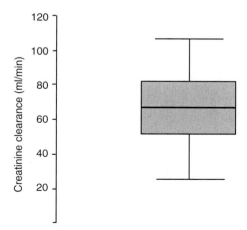

Figure 2.4 A box and whisker plot of creatinine clearance data in critically ill patients

References

1. Glantz SA. Biostatistics: how to detect, correct and prevent errors in the medical literature. *Circulation* 1980; **61**:1–7.
2. Altman DG. Statistics and ethics in medical research, v – analysing data. *BMJ* 1980; **281**:1473–1475.
3. Horan BF. Standard deviation, or standard error of the mean? [editorial] *Anaesth Intensive Care* 1982; **10**:297.
4. Avram MJ, Shanks CA, Dykes MHM *et al.* Statistical methods in anesthesia articles: an evaluation of two American journals during two six-month periods. *Anesth Analg* 1985; **64**:607–611.
5. Altman DG, Bland JM. The normal distribution. *BMJ* 1995; **310**:298.
6. Bland JM, Altman DG. Transforming data. *BMJ* 1996:**312**:770.
7. Altman DG, Gardner MJ. Presentation of variability. *Lancet* 1986; **ii**:639.

3

Principles of probability and inference

Samples and populations	Confidence intervals
Inferential statistics	Sample size and power calculations
–definition of probability	Parametric and non-parametric tests
–null hypothesis	Permutation tests
–P value	Bayesian inference
–type I and type II error	

Key points
- A sample is a group taken from a population.
- Data from samples are analysed to make inferences about the population.
- The null hypothesis states that there is no difference between the population variables in question.
- A type I or α error is where one rejects the null hypothesis incorrectly.
- A type II or β error is where one accepts the null hypothesis incorrectly.
- The P value is the probability of the event occurring by chance if the null hypothesis is true.
- A confidence interval indicates where the true population parameter probably lies.
- Power is the likelihood of detecting a difference between groups if one exists.
- Sample size is determined by α, β, Δ (delta, the difference between groups) and σ^2 (variance).

Samples and populations

A **sample** is a group taken from a **population.** The population may be all human beings on the earth, or just within a specific country, or all patients with a specific condition. A population may also consist of laboratory animals or cell types. A population, therefore, is not defined by geography, but by its characteristics. Examples of populations studied in anaesthesia include:

1. All day stay surgical patients undergoing general anaesthesia
2. Low-risk coronary artery bypass graft surgery patients
3. Critically ill patients in ICU with septic shock
4. Women undergoing caesarean section under spinal anaesthesia
5. Skeletal muscle fibres (from quadriceps muscle biopsy)

A clinical trial involves selecting a sample of patients, in the belief that the sample represents the response of the average patient in the population. Therefore, when applying the results of a trial to your practice, it remains important first to decide if the patients recruited in the trial (the trial 'sample') are similar to those that you wish to apply the results to (your clinical practice 'population').

Clear description and consideration of **inclusion** and **exclusion criteria** are therefore required.

Sample data are estimates of population parameters. Sampling procedures are therefore very important when selecting patients for study, so that they ultimately represent the population. Two common methods are to sequentially select all patients until the required number is obtained, or to randomly select (this is preferable) from a larger population. If patients are selected by other criteria, then it may **bias** the sample, such that it does not truly represent the population. In general, the larger the sample size, the more representative it will be of the population, but this involves more time and expense.

Inferential statistics

Inferential statistics is that branch of statistics where data are collected and analysed from a sample to make inferences about the larger population. The purpose is to derive an estimate of one or more population parameters, so that one may answer questions or test **hypotheses**.

The deductive philosophy of science attributes man with an inquiring mind that asks questions about himself and the environment. Each question is refined to produce a specific hypothesis and logical implications of the hypothesis that can be specifically tested. A scientific method is used to collect evidence, either by observation or controlled experiment, to try to support or refute the hypothesis.

Hypothesis tests are thus procedures for making rational decisions about the reality of observed effects. Most decisions require that an individual select a single choice from a number of alternatives. The decision is usually made without knowing whether or not it is absolutely correct. A rational decision is characterized by the use of a procedure which ensures that a probability of success is incorporated into the decision-making process. The procedure is strictly proscribed so that another individual, using the same information, would make the same decision.

The effects under study may be quantitative or qualitative, and can be summarized as various statistics (differences between means, contingency tables, correlation coefficients, etc.), each requiring an appropriate hypothesis testing procedure.

In logic, it is preferable to refute a hypothesis rather than try to prove one. The reason for this is that it is deductively valid to reject a hypothesis if the testable implications are found to be false (a method of argument known as *modus tollens*), but it is not deductively valid to accept a hypothesis if the testable implications are found to be true (known as the *fallacy of affirming the consequent*).

The specific implications may be found true (because of other circumstances) even though the general hypothesis may be false. Hypotheses may however be generally accepted based on weight of supporting evidence and lack of contrary evidence. A hypothesis can be supported by showing that an alternate mutually exclusive hypothesis is false.

Unlike logic, many of our real-world hypotheses cannot be definitively shown to be true or false. It is impossible to know everything about the universe. However it is possible to make predictions and make decisions. We accept hypotheses that are more likely. **Probability** is a theory of uncertainty that is used as a rational means of dealing with an uncertain world.

The meaning of the term probability depends upon one's philosophical orientation. In the classical approach, probabilities refer to the relative frequency of an event, if the experiment was repeated identically an infinite number of times. An example is the probability of getting a 6 if a die is rolled. In the subjective approach, the term probability refers to a degree of belief. This is perhaps more closely related to clinical research where one might consider for example the probability of death, an experiment that cannot be repeated an infinite number of times for any individual.

Probabilities are numbers ranging from 0 to 1.0 that are associated with the likelihood of events. A probability, $P(\text{event}) = 0$, means that the event is impossible, $P(\text{event}) = 1.0$ means that the event is certain. Most events have probabilities between these two extremes and there are mathematical rules governing probabilities.

For example, the probability of two or more independent events occurring is the sum of the individual probabilities. With a die the probability of rolling a 1 or a 2 on a single throw, $P(1 \text{ or } 2)$, is the sum of $P(1)$ and $P(2)$, or $2/6$. Thus, $P(1 \text{ or } 2) = 0.333$.

As an example of the scientific method of hypothesis testing, we can consider a drug trial, a controlled experiment designed to answer a question about some effect of a drug, either compared with placebo or another drug. Rather than try to prove directly that the drug causes a certain effect, the researcher tests whether or not the converse is likely. The converse is known as the **null hypothesis** (H_0), that the drug has no significant effect on some variable of interest, e.g. mean heart rate. The complementary **alternative hypothesis** (H_1) in this case is that the drug does cause some effect on mean heart rate.

Although we are interested in the effect of the drug in the population, we can only test the hypothesis in a subset of the population (**sample**), and then make inferences about the effect in the **population**. More specifically, the H_0 states that there is no difference in the variable of interest in the population from which the sample was drawn, compared with the control or other populations.

Thus the H_0 is mathematically written using the symbols for population parameters $H_0: \mu_1 = \mu_2$, where μ_1 and μ_2 are the mean heart rates in the two populations from which the samples are drawn.

To test the H_0, the variable of interest is measured in the sample after drug treatment, and data are analysed using an appropriate **significance test** from which a **test statistic** is derived (t, χ^2, F, etc.). The test statistic will have a sampling distribution that comprises all the possible values for the test statistic calculated from samples of the same size drawn randomly from the population. Each value of the test statistic will be associated with a certain probability, *P*, also known as the **P value**, which indicates the likelihood that the result obtained, or one more extreme, could have occurred randomly by chance, assuming that H_0 is true.

If *P* is less than an arbitrarily chosen value, known as α or the **significance level**, the H_0 is rejected. However the H_0 may be incorrectly rejected and this is known as a making a **type I error**. By convention, the α value is often set at 0.05 which means that one accepts a 5% probability of making a type I error. Other values for α can be chosen, depending on circumstances.

Note that if multiple comparisons are made, then there is increased likelihood of a type I error: the more you look for a difference, the more likely you are of finding one, even by chance (see Chapter 11)!

A **type II error** occurs when one accepts the H_0 incorrectly and the probability of this occurring is termed β. This will be discussed later when we talk about power.

Having rejected the H_0, it is usual to accept the complementary alternative hypothesis (H_1), in this case that the drug does cause some effect, (although strictly speaking we have not logically proved the H_1 or asserted that it is in fact true). We accept the H_1 but should remember that this is specifically for the experimental conditions of the trial and the sample tested. It is hoped that the results are **generalizable** to the population. However, it is up to the researchers and readers to decide whether or not this is valid.

In the example above, H_1 is that there is a difference in mean heart rate. The drug effect could be either to increase or decrease heart rate. This is known as a **two-tailed** hypothesis and the two-tailed form of the significance test is used. We can just be interested in one direction of effect, for example that the drug increases heart rate. In this case the complementary H_0 would state that these is no *increase* in heart rate, and a **one-tailed** test is used.

The two-tailed test is so named because when we specify an α of 0.05 in a two-tailed hypothesis, we are interested in results similar to or more extreme than that observed (with no indication of direction). Thus we are using the extremes at both ends or tails of the distribution, each tail containing half the total α probability, in this case, 2.5%.

A one-tailed test at an α of 0.05 would use just one end of the distribution and use different **critical values** to compare against the test statistic. Two-tailed tests should usually be used unless there are clear reasons specified in advance as to why one-tailed tests are appropriate for that study.[1]

We must remember that, based on our experiment, we make an inference based on likelihood. A statistically significant result may or may not be real because it is possible to make type I and type II errors. However, even if the result is real, we still need to decide whether or not the result is important. A very small effect may be real and shown to be statistically significant, but may also be clinically unimportant or irrelevant. The important finding is the likely size of the treatment effect (see Chapter 11).

Some investigators conduct trials and report only the result of significance tests; the null hypothesis is rejected, a real effect is observed and a P value is given indicating that the probability of this effect occurring by chance is very low.

However, the use of only P values has been criticized because they do not give an indication of the magnitude of any observed differences and thus no indication of the clinical significance of the result. Confidence intervals are often preferred when presenting results because they also provide this additional information.[2]

Confidence intervals

When estimating any population parameter by taking measurements from a sample, there is always some imprecision expected from the estimate. It is obviously helpful to give some measure of this imprecision.

There is an increasing tendency to quote **confidence intervals** (CI), either with P values or instead of them. This is preferable as it gives the reader a better idea of clinical applicability. If the 95% CI describing the difference between two mean values includes the point zero (i.e. zero difference), then obviously $P > 0.05$.

A 95% CI for any estimate gives a 95% probability that the true population parameter will be contained within that interval. Any % CI can be calculated, although 95% and 99% are the most common. CIs can be calculated for many statistics such as mean, median, proportion, odds ratio, slope of a regression line, etc.[2,3]

For example, in a study comparing the dose requirements for thiopentone in pregnant and non-pregnant patients,[4] the ED_{50} (95% CI) for hypnosis in the pregnant group was 2.6 (2.3–2.8) mg/kg. Thus we can be 95% certain that the true population ED_{50} is some value between 2.3 and 2.8 mg/kg. In addition, the pregnant to non-pregnant relative median potency (95% CI) for hypnosis was 0.83 (0.67–0.96). Because the 95% CI does not contain 1.0, we conclude that there is a significant difference in median potency between the two groups.

The lowest and highest values of the CI are also known as the lower and upper **confidence limits**.

It is commonly thought that the 95% CI for the population mean is the sample mean $\pm$ (1.96 $\times$ SEM), where SEM is the **standard error of the mean**. However this is only true for large sample sizes. If the sample size is small, the *t* **distribution** is applicable (see Chapter 5) and the 95% CI for the sample mean in small samples is calculated as the mean of the sample $\pm$ (the appropriate *t* value corresponding to 95% $\times$ SEM).

CI can be used to indicate the precision of any estimate. Obviously the smaller the CI the more precisely we assume the sample estimate represents the true population value. CI can also be used for hypothesis testing.

For example, if the CI for the difference between two means contains zero, then one can conclude that there is no significant difference between the two populations from which the samples were drawn at the significance % of the CI. Thus if we use a 95% CI, this is similar to choosing an α value of 0.05.

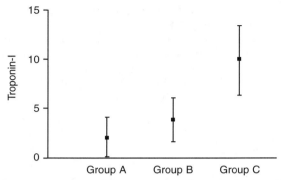

Figure 3.1 Theoretical plots of the mean and 95% confidence intervals (CIs) for troponin-I levels ($\mu g/l$) in three patient groups after major surgery. The 95% CI of group C do not overlap those of groups A and B, and so the difference in means is statistically significant ($P < 0.05$). The 95% CI of group B overlaps the mean value of group A and so it is not statistically significantly different (at $P < 0.05$)

It is possible to graphically illustrate the use of CI for hypothesis testing in a limited manner (Figure 3.1). If we show three sample means and their respective CIs, there is a significant difference between the group means if the respective CIs do not overlap. There is no difference if one CI includes the mean of the other sample. However, if the CIs just overlap, it is not easy to determine graphically whether or not there is a statistical difference between means and a statistical test is used.

For example, in a study comparing propofol requirements in normal patients with that in patients with small and large brain tumours,[5] the dose–response curves show that the 95% CIs for the control and small brain tumour contain the ED_{50} for the other group (Figure 3.2). There is thus no difference in ED_{50} for these two groups. However, these 95% CIs do not overlap the 95% CI for the large tumour group and so there is a difference in the ED_{50} of the large tumour group compared with the other two. Note however that there is overlap of the 95% CI for the ED_{95} and it is not clear from the graph whether or not this represents a significant difference. In this example, the authors also used a statistical test of significance.[5]

CIs can indicate statistical significance but, more importantly, by illustrating the accuracy of the sample estimates, presenting the results in the original units of measurement and showing the magnitude of any effect, they reveal more information. This enables the investigator (or reader) to determine whether or not any difference shown is *clinically* significant.

Sample size and power calculations

The difference between a sample mean and population mean is the **sampling error**. A larger sample size will decrease the sampling error.

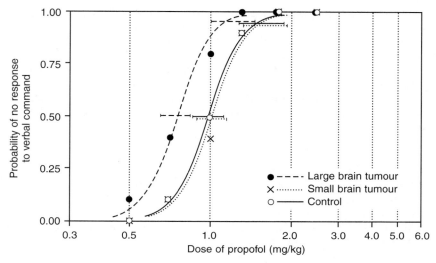

Figure 3.2 Calculated dose–response curves (log dose scale) for loss of response to verbal command in patients with brain tumour and patients undergoing non–cranial surgery. The 95% confidence intervals for the ED_{50} and ED_{95} are also displayed, slightly offset for clarity. Fraction of patients (out of ten) who failed to respond to verbal command are shown as (•) for patients with large brain tumour, (X) for patients with small tumour and (○) for control patients (From Chan *et al.* [5])

When designing a trial, two important questions are:

1. How large a sample is needed to allow statistical judgments that are accurate and reliable
2. How likely is a statistical test able to detect effects of a given size in a particular situation

Earlier we mentioned that it was possible to reject the H_0 incorrectly (a type I error), or accept the H_0 incorrectly (a type II error). The investigator sets a threshold for both these errors, often 0.05 for the type I or α error, and between 0.05 and 0.20 for the type II or β error.

Power is the likelihood of detecting a specified difference if it exists and it is equal to $1-\beta$. For example, in a paper comparing the duration of mivacurium neuromuscular block in normal and postpartum patients,[6] **power analysis** ($\beta = 0.1$, $\alpha = 0.05$) indicated that a sample size of 11 would be sufficient to detect a three-minute difference in clinical duration of neuromuscular block.

Performing power analysis and sample size estimation is an important aspect of experimental design,[7,8] because without these calculations sample size may be too large or too small. If sample size is too small, the experiment will lack the precision to provide reliable answers to the questions being investigated. If sample size is too large, time and resources will be wasted, often for minimal gain.

It is considered unethical to conduct a trial with low power because it wastes time and resources while subjecting patients to risk. The simplest way to increase power in a study is to increase the sample size, but power is only one of the factors that determine sample size.

There are various formulae for sample size depending on the study design and whether one is looking for difference in means, proportions, or other statistics.[7,9] Nomograms[8] and computer programs are also available.

As an example, if one is interested in calculating the sample size for a two-sided study comparing the means of two populations, then the following approximate formula can be used:[9]

$$n > \frac{2(z_{1-\alpha/2} + z_{1-\beta})^2 \, \sigma^2}{\Delta^2}$$

where n = the sample size required for each group, $z_{1-\alpha/2}$ = the value for the standard normal distribution for the $100(1-\alpha/2)$ percentile, $z_{1-\beta}$ = the value for the standard normal distribution for the $100(1-\beta)$ percentile, Δ = the effect size, or difference, that one wishes to detect, and σ^2 = the variance in the underlying populations.

Useful values for a two-sided study are:

if $\alpha = 0.05$, then $z_{1-\alpha/2} = 1.96$;   if $\alpha = 0.01$, then $z_{1-\alpha/2} = 2.58$
if $\beta = 0.20$, then $z_{1-\beta} = 0.84$;   if $\beta = 0.10$, then $z_{1-\beta} = 1.28$

It is evident that the sample size depends on these four factors:

1. Value chosen for α: a smaller α means a larger sample size
2. Value chosen for β: smaller β (higher power) means larger sample size
3. Δ (effect size): smaller Δ means larger sample size
4. σ^2 (variance) in the underlying populations: larger σ^2 means larger sample size

When using the sample size formula, the investigator can choose α, β and Δ.

Traditionally, many researchers choose $\beta = 0.2$, but this implies that the study only has 80% power (1 – 0.2), i.e. an 80% probability to detect a difference if one exists. Why should we accept a lower probability for α, typically 0.05, than β? Is it more important to protect against a type I or type II error? It has been argued that we should be more concerned about type I error because rejecting the H_0 would mean that we are accepting an effect and may incorrectly decide to implement a new therapy. It is generally important not to do this lightly.

Committing a type II error and concluding falsely that there is no effect will only delay the implementation of a new treatment (although this presupposes that some satisfactory alternative exists). However both errors are important and α and β values should be considered carefully, depending on the hypothesis being tested.

Delta (Δ), the effect size, is the difference that one wishes to detect. It is more difficult to detect a small difference than a large difference. Here the investigator is called upon to decide what is a *clinically significant* difference. This is arbitrary but should be plausible and acceptable by most peers.

For example, a muscle relaxant may truly increase serum potassium by 0.05 mmol/l. However we may decide that a clinically significant increase in potassium is 0.3 mmol/l. Thus the sample size is set so that a rise of 0.3 mmol/l is detectable. In this case, we may well fail to detect the true increase in serum potassium, but this is inconsequential because a rise of 0.05 mmol/l is not important. We have not however committed a type II error because the H_0 was that there is no difference as great as 0.3 mmol/l.

In another example, comparing postoperative morphine requirements after ketamine induction compared with thiopentone induction,[10] the effect size chosen was a 40% decrease in 24-hour morphine consumption. This was the expected effect size from a previous study in a different population. This effect was thought to be clinically relevant, although the authors would not dispute that some others might consider 30% or 50% to be thresholds for clinical relevance. Given the historical variance in morphine requirement derived from their acute pain database, a sample size of 20 was eventually calculated at $\alpha = 0.05$ and $\beta = 0.2$.

The **effect size** can be related to the standard deviation (Δ/σ) and categorized as small (< 0.2), medium (0.2–0.5) or large (> 0.5).

σ^2, the **variance** in the underlying populations, is the only variable that the investigator cannot choose. An estimate for this can be obtained from pilot studies or other published data, if available. The greatest concern is that if the variance is underestimated, on completion of the study at the given sample size, the power of the study will be diminished and a statistically significant difference may not be found.

The variance can also be minimized by maximizing measurement precision. For example, estimation of cardiac output using the thermo-dilution method has been shown to be more precise using measurements in triplicate and with iced injectate.[11,12] Thus, inclusion of these thermodilution methods in the study design can reduce the study cardiac output variance, and so limit the sample size required.

Note from the above formula that if one chooses Δ equal to σ, these two would then cancel mathematically in the sample size formula. However this is not a recommended technique for calculating sample size when one does not have an estimate of σ.

Having calculated a sample size, one usually increases the number by a factor based on projected dropouts from the study, and allowing for a reasonable margin of error in the estimate of σ. It is useful to recalculate sample size for greater estimates of σ because at times a surprisingly large sample size is required for a small change in σ and the feasibility of the whole study may be in doubt.

Sample size estimations for numerical data assume a normal distribution and so if the study data are skewed or non-parametric it is common to increase the sample size estimate by at least 10%.

The sample size formula for a two-sided comparison of proportions is:[9]

$$n > \frac{(z_{1-\alpha/2} + z_{1-\beta})^2(p_1q_1 + p_2q_2)}{\Delta^2}$$

where n = the sample size required for each group, $z_{1-\alpha/2}$ = the value for the standard normal distribution for the $100(1-\alpha/2)$ percentile, $z_{1-\beta}$ = the value for the standard normal distribution for the $100(1-\beta)$ percentile, p_1

and p_2 = the expected proportions in the two groups, q_1 and q_2 =1-p_1 and 1-p_2, respectively, Δ = the effect size, which is p_1-p_2.

Thus, the sample size for a difference in proportions depends on four factors:

1. Value chosen for α: a smaller α means a larger sample size
2. Value chosen for β: smaller β (higher power) means larger sample size
3. Δ (effect size, p_1–p_2): smaller Δ means larger sample size
4. Number of study endpoints (p_1): rare events require larger sample size

There may also be several outcomes of interest and the sample size calculations for each of these outcomes may be different. Good trial design dictates that the sample size should be based on the **primary endpoint**, though it may be further increased if important secondary endpoints are also being studied.

Although a sample size is calculated, *a priori*, before the study begins, it is also useful to use the same formula to calculate the power of the study, *a posteriori*, after the study has been completed. This can be useful when the H_0 is accepted because it indicates how likely a given difference could have been detected using the actual standard deviation from the final study samples, rather than the original estimate.

Previous authors have noted that many published studies had failed to study an adequate number of patients, such that they were unlikely to have reliably determined a true treatment effect if it existed.[7–9,13,14] This has been a common error in anaesthesia studies (see Chapter 11).

Parametric and non-parametric tests

In the previous discussion of statistical inference and hypothesis testing, it was necessary to determine the probability of any observed difference. This probability is based on the sampling distribution of a test statistic. It is important to realize that there are assumptions made when using these test statistics (see also Chapters 5 and 6).

Parametric tests are based on estimates of parameters. In the case of normally distributed data, the tests are based on sampling distributions derived from μ or σ. Parametric tests are based on the actual magnitude of values (quantitative, continuous data), and can only be used for data on a numerical scale (cardiac output, renal blood flow, etc.). The parametric tests discussed later in this book have many inherent assumptions and thus should only be used when these are met.

Non-parametric tests were developed for situations when the researcher knows nothing about the parameters of the variable of interest in the population.[15] Non-parametric methods do not rely on the estimation of parameters (such as the mean or the standard deviation). Non-parametric tests should generally be used to analyse ordinal and categorical data (rating of patient satisfaction, incidence of adverse events, etc.).

A common criticism of non-parametric tests is that they are not as powerful as parametric tests. This means that they are not as likely to detect a significant difference as parametric tests, if the conditions of the parametric test are fulfilled. When the parametric assumptions are not met, non-parametric tests often become more powerful.[15]

Proponents of parametric tests agree that non-parametric methods are most appropriate when the sample sizes are small. However, the tests of significance of many of the non-parametric statistics described here are based on asymptotic (large sample) theory and meaningful tests often cannot be performed if the sample sizes become too small (say, $n < 10$). When the data set is large (say, $n > 100$), it often makes little sense to use non-parametric statistics because the sample means will follow the normal distribution even if the respective variable is not normally distributed in the population, or is not measured very well. This is a result of an extremely important principle called the **central limit theorem**.

The central limit theorem states that, as the sample size increases, the shape of the sampling distribution approaches normal shape, even if the distribution of the variable in question is not normal. For $n = 30$, the shape of that distribution is 'almost' normal. Ordinal data can be analysed with parametric tests in large samples, particularly if the sample data represent a population variable on a continuous scale.[16]

Proponents of the non-parametric tests argue that the power of these tests is very close to the parametric tests even when all conditions for the parametric test are satisfied. When the parametric assumptions are not met, non-parametric tests actually become more powerful. Power efficiency is the increase in sample size necessary to make the test as powerful at an alpha level and given sample size. Asymptotic relative efficiency is the same concept for large sample sizes, and is independent of the type I error. The power for the common non-parametric tests is often 95% of the equivalent parametric test.[15]

Permutation tests[17,18]

There has been renewed interest in a third approach for testing significance, apart from using the common parametric and non-parametric statistics. One important assumption of statistical inference is that the samples are drawn randomly from the population. In reality, this is almost never the case. Our samples are mostly not truly random samples from the population but are instead comprised only of subjects to which we have access and are then able to recruit. Thus the subjects who enter a trial conducted in a hospital will depend on many geographical and social as well as medical factors influencing admissions to a particular hospital. In almost all clinical trials, we actually study a non-random sample of the population that undergoes random allocation to treatments. It could be argued then that the results of the trial cannot be generalized to the population at large and it is inappropriate to determine the probability of any differences based on sampling theory from the population.[17,18]

An alternative **permutation test** works out all the possible outcomes given your sample size, determines the likelihood of each of them and then calculates how likely it is to have achieved the given result or one more extreme.

As a simple example, consider tossing a coin six times to determine whether or not the coin was biased. If the outcome of interest is the number of heads, the probabilities range from: $P(0$ heads$)$ to $P(6$ heads$)$. We can thus work out the probability of getting a result as extreme as 1 head by $P(0$ heads$) + P(1$ head$) + P(5$ heads$) + P(6$ heads$) = 14/64$! This being greater than an arbitrary P value of 0.05 would lead us to conclude that the coin was not biased. However if we got 0 heads, the probability of a result this extreme is $P(0$ heads$) + P(6$ heads$) = 2/64$, that is less than an arbitrary P value of 0.05 would lead us to conclude that the coin was biased. Note that we have used a two-tailed hypothesis in these examples.

Thus the permutation tests provide a result exactly applicable to the samples under study and make no assumptions about the distribution of the underlying (and remaining) population. We are however usually interested in generalizing our specific sample results to the population and it appears that permutation tests do not permit this. However, if other researchers replicate the trial with different samples and achieve similar conclusions, then the weight of evidence would lend us to support (or reject) the overall hypothesis.

The only permutation test in common use is **Fisher's exact test** (Chapter 6). This is because the permutations are very time intensive and only recently has the advent of personal computers made these tests more feasible.

Bayesian inference

Use of **P value** to determine whether an observed effect is statistically significant has its critics.[19,22] This is because a P value is a mathematical statement of probability; it both ignores how large is the **treatment effect**, and conclusions based solely on it do not take into consideration prior knowledge. Thus, an observed effect that is not statistically significant, but is consistent with previous study results, is more likely to be true than a similar treatment effect observed that had not been previously reported.

Clinicians do not consider a trial result in isolation. They generally consider what is already known and judge whether the new trial information modifies their belief and practice. This is one explanation why clinicians may reach different conclusions from the same study data.

A Bayesian approach incorporates prior knowledge in its conclusion.[20–22] It has been developed from **Bayes' theorem**[*], a formula used to calculate the probability of an outcome, given a positive test result (see Chapter 8). It combines the **prior probability** and the study P value, to calculate a **posterior probability**.

For example, if a new alpha$_2$-agonist is tested to see if it reduces the rate of myocardial ischaemia, it would be a plausible hypothesis because of what is known about other alpha$_2$-agonists. The resultant P value is

---

[*]Thomas Bayes (1763): 'An essay towards solving a problem in the doctrine of chances'.

0.04. There are two possible explanations for this result. Either, it was a chance finding (1 in 25) or it was a true effect of the new drug. The second option makes much more sense because of prior knowledge (this would still be the case if the *P* value was 0.06).

Alternatively, if the same study also found that the new alpha$_2$-agonist reduced the rate of vomiting ($P = 0.04$), this would be more likely to be a chance finding. This is because prior knowledge suggests that, if anything, other alpha$_2$-agonists increase the risk of nausea and vomiting.

Bayesian inference has appeal because it considers the totality of knowledge.[19-23] In fact, there are literally two opposing camps of statisticians: frequentists and Bayesianists!

One of the criticisms of Bayesian inference is that the methods used to determine prior probability are ill-defined.

References

1. Bland JM, Altman DG. One and two sided tests of significance. *Br Med J* 1994; **309**:248.
2. Gardner MJ, Altman DG. Confidence intervals rather than *P* values: estimation rather than hypothesis testing. *Br Med J* 1986; **292**:746–750.
3. Gardner MJ, Altman DG. Statistics with Confidence – Confidence Intervals and Statistical Guidelines. *British Medical Journal*, London, 1989.
4. Gin T, Mainland P, Chan MTV *et al.* Decreased thiopental requirements in early pregnancy. *Anesthesiology* 1997; **86**:73–78.
5. Chan MTV, Gin T, Poon WS. Propofol requirement is decreased in patients with large supratentorial brain tumor. *Anesthesiology* 1999; **90**:1571–1576.
6. Gin T, Derrick J, Chan MTV, *et al.* Postpartum patients have slightly prolonged neuromuscular block following mivacurium. *Anesth Analg* 1998; **86**:82–85.
7. Florey C du V. Sample size for beginners. *Br Med J* 1993; **306**:1181–1184.
8. Altman DG. Statistics and ethics in medical research. III How large a sample. *Br Med J* 1980; **281**:1336–1338.
9. Campbell MJ, Julious SA, Altman DG. Estimating sample sizes for binary, ordered categorical, and continuous outcomes in two group comparisons. *Br Med J* 1995; **311**:1145–1148.
10. Ngan Kee WD, Khaw KS, Ma ML *et al.* Postoperative analgesic requirement after cesarean section: a comparison of anesthetic induction with ketamine or thiopental. *Anesth Analg* 1997; **85**:1294–1298.
11. Stetz CW, Miller RG, Kelly GE *et al.* Reliability of the thermodilution method in determination of cardiac output in clinical practice. *Am Rev Respir Dis* 1982; **126**:1001–1004.
12. Bazaral MG, Petre L, Novoa R. Errors in thermodilution cardiac output measurements caused by rapid pulmonary artery temperature decreases after cardiopulmonary bypass. *Anesthesiology* 1992; **77**:31–37.
13. Goodman NW, Hughes AO. Statistical awareness of research workers in British anaesthesia. *Br J Anaesth* 1992; **68**:321–324.
14. Frieman JA, Chalmers TC, Smith H *et al.* The importance of beta, the type II error and sample size in the design and interpretation of the randomized controlled trial. *N Engl J Med* 1978; **299**:690–694.
15. Siegal S, Castellan NJ Jr. Nonparametric Statistics for the Behavioral Sciences. 2nd ed. McGraw-Hill, New York 1988.
16. Moses LE, Emerson JD, Hosseini H. Statistics in practice. Analyzing data from ordered categories. *N Engl J Med* 1984; **311**:442–448.

17. Ludbrook J. Advantages of permutation (randomization) tests in clinical and experimental pharmacology and physiology. *Clin Exp Pharmacol Physiol* 1994; **21**:673–686.
18. Ludbrook J, Dudley H. Issues in biomedical statistics: statistical inference. *Aust NZ J Surg* 1994; **64**:630–636.
19. Browner WS, Newman TB. Are all significant p values created equal? The analogy between diagnostic tests and clinical research. *JAMA* 1987; **257**:2459–2463.
20. Brophy JM, Joseph L. Bayesian interim statistical analysis of randomised trials. *Lancet* 1997; **349**:1166–1168.
21. Goodman SN. Towards evidence based medical statistics: the P value fallacy. *Ann Intern Med* 1999; **130**:995–1004.
22. Goodman SN. Towards evidence based medical statistics: the Bayes factor. *Ann Intern Med* 1999; **130**:1005–1013.
23. Davidoff F. Standing statistics right side up. *Ann Intern Med* 1999; **130**:1019–1021.

4

Research design

<table>
<tr>
<td>

Bias and confounding
   –randomization and stratification
Types of research design
   –observation vs. experimentation
   –case reports and case series
   –case-control study
   –cohort study
   –association vs. causation
   –randomized controlled trial
   –self-controlled and crossover trials

</td>
<td>

Randomization techniques
   –block randomization
   –stratification
   –minimization
Blinding
Sequential analysis
Interim analysis
Data accuracy and data checking
Missing data
Intention to treat

</td>
</tr>
</table>

Key points
- Bias is a systematic deviation from the truth.
- Randomization and blinding reduce bias.
- Confounding occurs when another factor also affects the outcome of interest.
- Observational studies may be retrospective, cross-sectional or prospective.
- The gold standard study is a double-blind randomized controlled trial (RCT).
- Sequential analysis (interim analysis) allows the early stopping of a trial as soon as a significant difference is identified.
- Analysis of patients in an RCT should be by 'intention to treat'.

In the past, large dramatic advances in medicine (e.g. discovery of ether anaesthesia) did not require a clinical trial to demonstrate benefit. Most current advances have small-to-moderate benefits, and a reliable method of assessment is required to demonstrate a true effect.

Bias and confounding

In a research study, an observed difference between groups may be a result of treatment effect (a true difference), random variation (chance), or a deficiency in the research design which enabled systematic differences to exist in either the group characteristics, measurement, data collection or analysis.[1] These deficiencies lead to **bias**, a systematic deviation from the truth. There are many potential sources of bias in medical research. Examples include:

1. Selection bias – where group allocation leads to a spurious improved outcome because one group is healthier or at lower risk than another
2. Detection bias – where measurements or observations in one group are not as vigilantly sought as in the other
3. Observer bias – where the person responsible for data collection is able to use their judgment as to whether an event occurred or not, or determine its extent

3. Reporting bias (or recall bias) – where a person's group identity influences their likelihood of accurately reporting previous experiences, symptoms or outcome
5. Response bias – where patients who enroll in a trial differ from those in the population of interest (and so the results may not be generally applicable)
6. Publication bias – where negative studies are less likely to be submitted, or accepted, for publication

Bias is **systematic error**. Other sources of variability in clinical research are **random errors**, and these can be managed by studying large numbers of patients. Systematic error cannot be compensated for by increasing sample size.

Studies are often performed on groups of patients with special characteristics, by interested clinicians. The actual process of study – patient explanation, informed consent, measurement, and follow-up – may result in more favourable outcomes in such patients. This process is known as the **Hawthorne effect**, a type of bias. It can be reduced by masking the actual intent of the study or by including a suitable control group for comparison (or demonstration that bias has not occurred to any significant extent). The two most important features of trial design that reduce bias are randomization and blinding (see below).

Confounding occurs when baseline characteristics of the groups being compared are unequally distributed and this also has an effect on the outcome of interest. In this situation it becomes difficult to attribute differences in eventual outcome to a treatment effect, as they cannot easily be separated from the confounding. Such baseline characteristics are called confounding factors or covariates. Note that a confounding factor must be both unequally distributed between groups at baseline *and* have an effect on the outcome of interest (if there is no inequality, then the effect of the factor will be equalized between groups). Examples of possible confounding factors include gender, age, pre-existing health (or risk) status and myocardial function (Table 4.1). Confounding can be reduced by increasing the size of the trial and using randomization, so that, on average, all possible confounding factors will be evenly distributed between groups. Confounding can also be specifically minimized by stratifying randomization (see below) or by 'adjustment' using multivariate statistical techniques (see Chapters 6 and 8).[2]

Types of research design

Research may involve observation or experimentation. Observational studies have no stipulated interventions, but follow a patient's natural progress over a period of time and events of interest are recorded (such as patient characteristics, occurrence and incidence of complications, hospital readmission rate, and death). The clinical significance of such outcomes may then be considered; this is usually achieved by comparison with either a preconceived expected rate of events, or with some other reference group. This process is open to many types of bias,

Table 4.1 Examples of possible confounding factors in clinical research. Confounding occurs when baseline characteristics of the groups being compared are both unequally distributed and have an effect on the outcome of interest

Outcome of interest	Possible confounder	Explanation
Postoperative emesis	Gender	Women have a higher incidence of postoperative nausea and vomiting
Postoperative opioid requirement	Patient age	Opioid requirement decreases with age
ICU mortality	APACHE III score	Baseline predictor of mortality
Duration of ICU stay	LV function	Poor LV function is associated with increased complication rate (gas exchange, inotrope requirement, renal function, sepsis)
Perioperative blood loss	Previous cardiac surgery	Increased bleeding due to adhesions, increased thrombolysis, prolonged duration of surgery

for example selection bias, recall bias and detection bias.[1] Therefore care must be taken if observational studies are to yield reliable results.

Observational studies may be retrospective, cross-sectional or prospective. Retrospective studies look backwards in time and record events that have already occurred. Such studies are particularly exposed to bias, as data may be incomplete, inaccurate or selectively retrieved. A **cross-sectional study** records observations at a specific point in time and is often used to establish prevalence rates or provide other descriptive data. A survey is a typical cross-sectional study; in order to be confident that the surveyed sample accurately represents the population, the response rate should exceed 70% (ideally > 95%). A prospective study looks forward in time, and so can be pre-planned, maximizing data accuracy and potentially used to test an intervention (an experiment, or trial).

An experimental research design includes an intervention and is the best method to evaluate an established treatment or to investigate the potential benefits of a proposed new treatment. A **clinical trial** uses humans as the experimental subjects.

Case reports and case series

These observational studies report on various patient and perioperative characteristics in a single patient or patient group of interest. They have some value in reporting how patients respond under certain circumstances. Descriptive information, such as patient response, complications and outcome, can support a proposed treatment plan. However because there is no control group, conclusions concerning the relative efficacy of a treatment are weak. For example, if a unit reports outstanding success with a new nutritional regimen in patients undergoing major surgery, these benefits may be caused by other factors, such as their actual patient population (perhaps low risk), excellent surgical or anaesthetic techniques, or other aspects of the patients' perioperative care. Ideally such reports should only be used to generate hypotheses that should then be tested with more advanced research designs.

Case-control study

A case-control study is an observational study that begins with a definition of the outcome of interest and then looks backward in time to identify possible exposures, or risk factors, associated with that outcome (Figure 4.1).[3] Patients who experienced this outcome are defined as **'cases'**; patients who did not are defined as **'controls'**. This study design is particularly useful for uncommon events, as cases can be collected over a long period of time (retrospective and prospective) or from specialist units which have a higher proportion of patients with these outcomes. The case-control study has been under-utilized in anaesthesia and intensive care research. It should become more popular as large departmental and institutional databases are established, thereby allowing exploratory studies to be undertaken.

In most case-control studies the control patients are matched to the cases on some criteria, usually age and gender. The aim of this **matching** process is to equalize some baseline characteristics so that confounding is reduced. This allows a more precise estimate of the effect of various exposures of interest. It is important to understand that matched

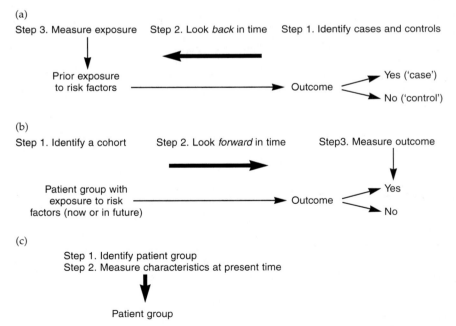

Figure 4.1 Types of observational studies: (a) case-control study; (b) cohort study; (c) cross-sectional study

characteristics cannot then be compared, because they will have equal values for cases and controls! Another way of reducing the effects of confounding is to use multivariate statistical adjustment (see Chapter 8). It is common to increase the sample size of a case-control study by using a higher proportion of controls than cases. Hence 1:2, 1:3 or 1:4 matching is commonly used.

Once the cases and controls have been selected, the aim is to look *back in time* at specific exposures that may be related to the outcome of interest. The exposures may include patient characteristics (such as severity of illness, pre-existing disease, age group* or smoking status), drug administration, and type of surgery (or surgeon!). In order to minimize bias, the definition of each of these exposures should be defined before the data are collected and efforts used to acquire them should be equivalent for cases and controls.[3]

Rebollo *et al.*[4] investigated possible factors that were associated with infection following cardiac surgery. Over a 12-month period they identified postoperative infection in 89 patients ('cases') and these were matched to 89 controls. They then retrospectively identified the following perioperative characteristics which were significantly associated with infection: patient age > 65 years, urgent surgery, prolonged surgery and use of blood transfusion.

Cohort study

A cohort study observes a group of patients *forward in time* in order to record their eventual outcome. A specific group of patients are identified (a '**cohort**'), and these can be matched to one or several other control groups for comparison (Figure 4.1). Because cohort studies are usually performed prospectively, the accuracy of the data can be improved and so results are generally accepted as being more reliable than in retrospective case-control studies.[5] But because the outcome of interest may occur infrequently, or take a long time to develop, this design may require a large number of patients to be observed over a long period of time in order to collect enough outcome events. A cohort study is therefore relatively inefficient.

Observational studies can be used to estimate the **risk** of an outcome in patients who are exposed to a risk factor versus those not exposed. In prospective cohort studies this is described by the **risk ratio** (also known as **relative risk**). If exposure is not associated with the outcome, the risk ratio is equal to one, if there is an increased risk, the risk ratio will be greater than one, and if there is a reduced risk, the risk ratio will be less than one. For example, if the risk ratio for smokers acquiring a postoperative wound infection is 10,[6] then smokers have a 10-fold increased risk of wound infection compared to non-smokers. If the risk ratio for men reporting postoperative emesis is 0.6, then men have a 40% reduction $(1.0 - 0.6 = 0.4)$ in postoperative emesis compared with women.

The risk ratio can be expressed with **95% confidence intervals** (CI).[7] If this interval does not include the value of one, the association between

---

*Only if age was not used to match cases and controls.

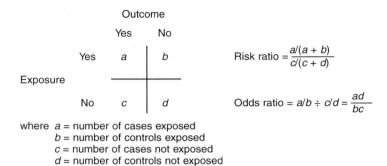

where a = number of cases exposed
b = number of controls exposed
c = number of cases not exposed
d = number of controls not exposed

Figure 4.2 In prospective cohort studies the risk ratio is equal to the risk of an outcome when exposed compared to the risk when not exposed. For case-control studies (outcome 'yes' = cases, outcome 'no' = controls), the value for the denominator is unreliable and so the odds ratio is used as an estimate of risk

exposure and outcome is significant (P < 0.05). Because accurate information concerning total numbers is unavailable in a retrospective case-control study (because sample size is set by the researcher), incidence rate and risk cannot be accurately determined, and the **odds ratio** is used as the estimate of risk (Figure 4.2). Odds ratios can also be expressed with 95% CI.[7] The statistical methods used to analyse case-control and comparative cohort studies are presented in more detail in Chapter 6.

An example of a case-control study by Myles *et al.*[8] was one designed to investigate the potential role of calcium antagonists and ACE inhibitors in causing persistent vasodilatation after cardiac surgery. Overall, 42 cases (patients with persistent low systemic vascular resistance) were identified in a 12-month period and these were matched for age and sex to 84 controls. Looking back at their preoperative medications ('exposure'), 11 cases and 19 controls had been given ACE inhibitors, and 22 cases and 62 controls had been given calcium antagonists. Univariate ('unadjusted') odds ratios were 1.21 and 0.39, respectively. These were 'adjusted' using a multivariate statistical technique in order to balance for possible confounding – there was no significant association for either ACE inhibitors (odds ratio 1.33, 95% CI: 0.53–3.34) or calcium antagonists (odds ratio 0.49, 95% CI: 0.21–1.13).

An example of a cohort study was one designed by Strom *et al.*,[9] who investigated the adverse effects of the non-steroidal drug, ketorolac, on postoperative outcome. They compared 10 272 patients who received ketorolac, and matched them to 10 247 treated with opiates, investigating the risk of gastrointestinal and operative site bleeding. The risk (odds) ratio of gastrointestinal bleeding in those exposed to ketorolac was 1.3 (or 30% greater risk), 95% CI: 1.11–1.52. This risk was increased in patients treated longer than 5 days, and in those over 70 years of age. Because their study design enabled them to include very large numbers of patients, they were able to give a precise estimate of risk (i.e. narrow 95%

CI). Nevertheless, because patients were not randomized to each treatment group (ketorolac or opiates), concern over potential bias and confounding remain.

Association vs. causation

Because observational studies do not require a specific intervention, and many departments and institutions now manage extensive patient databases, it is relatively easy to obtain information on large numbers of patients. Such studies form the basis of much epidemiological research ('study of the health of populations') and their value lies in their efficiency, in that 100s or 1000s of patients can be analysed. But it must be recognized that the results of observational studies depend heavily on the accuracy of the original data set ('gigo': garbage in, garbage out). Bias and confounding are difficult to avoid and should always be considered as alternative explanations to an observed relationship between drug exposure (or intervention) and outcome.

Even if a relationship between exposure and outcome is beyond doubt, it does not prove that exposure caused the outcome: 'association does not imply causation'. In order to demonstrate causation requires the collective weight of evidence from a number of potential sources.[5,10,11] All the available evidence should be processed:

1. Is the evidence consistent?
2. Is there a demonstrated temporal sequence between drug exposure and adverse outcome? This is particularly relevant for case-control studies and case reports.
3. Is there a dose–response relationship (greater risk if exposed to higher doses, or for longer periods)?
4. Is there biological plausibility?

It is the mounting body of supportive evidence that finally supports causation.

Randomized controlled trial

The gold standard experimental research design is the **prospective randomized controlled trial**. Here patients are allocated to a treatment group and their outcome is compared with a similar group allocated to an alternative treatment. This reference group is called the **control group** and its role is to represent an equivalent patient group who have not received the intervention of interest. A controlled trial therefore allows meaningful conclusions concerning the relative benefits (or otherwise) of the intervention of interest. There may be one or more control groups, consisting of patients who receive a current standard treatment or placebo.

A randomized controlled trial is sometimes referred to as a **parallel groups trial**, in that each group is exposed to treatment and then followed concurrently forwards in time to measure the relative effects of each treatment (Figure 4.3).

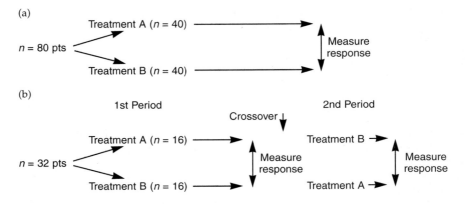

Figure 4.3 Comparing two treatments (A and B) with a standard parallel trial design or a crossover trial design: (a) parallel groups trial; (b) crossover trial

Trials which compare an active treatment to placebo can demonstrate whether the active treatment has some significant effect and/or to document the side-effects of that active treatment (relative to placebo). If the control group is to receive another active treatment (usually current standard treatment), then the aim of the trial is to demonstrate that the new treatment has a significant advantage over current treatment. This often has more clinical relevance.

For example, Suen *et al.*[12] enrolled 204 women undergoing laparoscopic gynaecological surgery and randomly allocated each to receive ondansetron or placebo, and measured the incidence of nausea and vomiting. Patients were followed up for 24 hours. The investigators clearly demonstrated that ondansetron was an effective anti-emetic in that it reduced emetic symptoms by approximately 50%.

Fujii *et al.*[13] randomized 100 women undergoing major gynaecolgical surgery into two groups (domperidone 20 mg, or granisetron 2 mg). They chose domperidone as the comparator because it was a commonly used anti-emetic. They clearly demonstrated that granisetron was more effective in their patient population. This provides additional, clinically useful information.

Self-controlled and crossover trials

It is difficult to detect a significant difference between groups in trials when the observation of interest is subject to a lot of variation ('background noise'). This **variance** can be reduced by restricting trial entry (excluding patients who have extreme values or who may react differently to the intervention) or by improving measurement precision. Stratification and blocking can be used to equalize potential confounding variables (see later).

Another way of reducing variance is to allow each patient to act as their own control and so all patient characteristics affecting the outcome of interest are equalized. This is a suitable design to test the effect of a new drug or treatment on a group of patients and is known as a **self-controlled**, or **before and after** study. Here, baseline measurements are taken, the treatment is then given and after an appropriate period of time measurements are repeated. Assuming that the patients were otherwise in a stable condition, then any change in the observation can be attributed to the effect of the treatment. The appropriate methods to analyse this 'paired' data are presented in Chapters 5 and 6.

When two or more interventions are to be compared in patients who act as their own control, they need to be exposed to each of the treatments. This requires they be crossed over from one treatment group to the next; this is known as a **crossover trial**.[14,15] This is best achieved by randomizing patients to each treatment, measuring the effect, and then giving them the alternative treatment, followed by another set of measurements (see Figure 4.4).

Crossover trials are most useful when assessing treatment for a stable disease, or where the intervention being tested has a short period of onset and offset and the effect can be measured quickly. Each treatment period can be separated by a '**washout period**', enabling the effect of the first treatment to dissipate before testing the second treatment.

This is a very powerful research design as it avoids the confounding effect of patient characteristics, thereby markedly reducing variance and maximizing the likelihood of detecting a treatment effect. It is a very efficient design: the sample size required to show a difference between groups can often be substantially reduced.

Nevertheless, readers must be aware of potential problems in using this design.[14,15] These include avoiding a **carry-over effect** (where the effects of the first treatment are still operating when the next treatment is evaluated), **period effect** (where there is a tendency for the group either to improve or deteriorate over time – the second treatment evaluation will be confounded by this) and **sequence effect** (where the order of treatments also has an effect on outcome). There are statistical methods available to investigate these effects.[14,15] Patient dropouts also have a potent adverse impact on study power (because each patient contributes data at all periods, for each treatment), and because each patient requires at least two treatments, trial duration usually needs to be extended. Despite these concerns, crossover trials are a very efficient method to compare interventions, when well designed and correctly analysed. If possible, the crossover point should be blinded to reduce bias.

In general, crossover trials have been under-utilized in anaesthesia research. If readers are considering employing a crossover trial design, we would recommend two excellent reviews.[14,15] Some examples can be found in the anaesthetic and intensive care literature.[16,17]

When interest is focused on one patient and their response to one or more treatments, this is known as an '**n-of-1 trial**'. This is usually performed in the setting of clinical practice when treating a specific patient (who may be resistant to standard treatment, or who warrants a new or experimental treatment).[18] The results are not intended to be generalized to other patients. Ideally, an *n*-of-1 trial should be performed under blinded conditions. This trial design may be useful when optimizing, say, an anaesthetic technique for a patient requiring repeated surgical procedures or a course of electroconvulsive therapy. It may also be used in intensive care, say to optimize a sedative or analgesic regimen for a problematic patient. Obviously the trial result will only apply to that patient, but this is a useful method of objectively measuring individual response to changes in treatment.

Randomization techniques

To minimize bias, the allocation of patients to each treatment group should be randomized. The commonest method is **simple randomization**, which allocates patients in such a way that each has an equal chance* of being allocated to any particular group and that process is not affected by previous allocations. This is usually guided by referring to a table of random numbers or a computer-generated list. This commonly used method has the value of simplicity, but may result in unequal numbers of patients allocated to each group or unequal distribution of potential confounding factors (particularly in smaller studies).

Block randomization is a method used to keep the number of patients in each group approximately the same (usually in blocks with random sizes of 4, 6 or 8). As each block of patients is completed, the number in each group will then be equal.

Stratification is a very useful method to minimize confounding.[2,19–21] The identified confounding factors act as criteria for separate randomization schedules, ensuring that the confounding variables are equalized between groups. Here, the presence of a confounding variable divides patients into separate blocks (with and without the confounder), and each block of patients is separately randomized into groups, so that ultimately equal numbers of patients with that particular confounder will be allocated to each group. This allows a clearer interpretation of the effect of an intervention on eventual outcome. Common stratifying variables include gender, patient age, risk strata, smoking status (these depend on whether it is considered they may have an effect on a particular outcome) and, for multi-centred research, each institution.

For example, in a study investigating the potential benefits of lung CPAP during cardiopulmonary bypass in patients undergoing cardiac surgery, Berry *et al.*[22] first stratified patients according to their preoperative ventricular function in order to balance out an important confounding factor known to have an effect on postoperative recovery. The patients were then randomly allocated into groups. This method resulted in near-equal numbers of patients in both groups having poor ventricular function (Figure 4.4).

A **Latin square design** is a more complex method to control for two or more confounding variables. Here the levels of each confounding

---

*In some trials there may intentionally be an uneven allocation to each treatment group, so that there is a fixed (known) chance other than 0.5. This is a valid method to increase the sample size of a particular group if its variance is to be more precisely estimated.

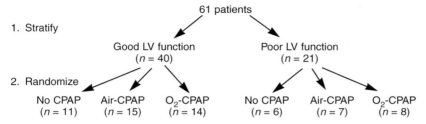

Figure 4.4 An example of stratified randomization adapted from Berry *et al.*[22] Here, patients are first stratified, or divided, into blocks (according to left ventricular function) and then separately randomized in order to equalize the numbers of patients in each group with poor ventricular function. This reduces confounding

variable make up the rows and columns of a square and patients are randomized to each treatment cell.[23]

Minimization is another method of equalizing baseline characteristics. Here the distribution of relevant patient (or other) factors between the groups is considered when the next patient is to be enrolled and group allocation is aimed at minimizing any imbalance. Minimization is a particularly useful method of group allocation when there is a wish to equalize groups for several confounding variables.[24]

Minimization also has advantages in situations where randomization is unacceptable because of ethical concerns (see Chapter 12).

However, because group allocation is no longer randomly determined, minimization may expose a trial to bias. For example, a selection bias may occur whereby 'sicker' patients are placed into a control group. A solution to this can be achieved by retaining random allocation, but modifying the ratio of random allocation (from 1:1 to, say, 1:4), to increase the chance the next patient will be allocated to the desired group.

Knowledge of group allocation should be kept secure (blind) until after the patient is enrolled in a trial. Prior knowledge may affect the decision to recruit a particular patient and so distort the eventual generalizability of the trial results. The commonest method is to use sealed, opaque envelopes.

Blinding

Blinding of the patient (**single-blind**), observer (**double-blind**), and investigator or person responsible for the analysis of results (sometimes referred to as **triple-blind**) can dramatically reduce bias. It is otherwise tempting for the subject or researcher to consciously or unconsciously distort observations, measurement, recordings, data cleaning or analyses.

In a case-control study, the person responsible for identification and recording of exposure should be blinded to group identity.[4] Similarly, in a comparative cohort study, the observer should be blinded to group identity when identifying and recording outcome events. In clinical trials, a double-blind design should be used whenever possible. If, because of the nature of the intervention, it is impossible to blind the observer or investigator, then a separate person who remains blinded to group identity should be responsible for identifying eventual outcome events. If a patient cannot be blinded to their treatment group, then outcome events should be objectively and clearly predetermined in order to reduce detection and reporting bias. Efforts made to maximize blinding in trial design are repaid by improved scientific credibility and enhanced impact on clinical practice.

Sequential analysis

If the results of a clinical trial are analysed and it is found that there is no significant difference between groups, then some investigators continue the trial in order to recruit more patients, hoping that the larger numbers will eventually result in statistical significance. This is grossly incorrect.[23] Some investigators do not even report that they have done this and so the reader remains unaware of this potent source of bias. The more 'looks' at the data, the greater the chance of a **type I error** (i.e. falsely rejecting the null hypothesis and concluding that a difference exists between groups).[25–30]

Sequential analysis is a collection of valid statistical methods used to repeatedly compare the outcome of two groups while a trial is in progress.[26] This allows a clinical trial to be stopped as soon as a significant difference between groups is identified. This is a useful trial design to investigate rare conditions, as the traditional randomized controlled trial could take a very long time to recruit sufficient numbers of patients, or would need to be multi-centred (and this requires much greater effort to establish and run). Sequential analysis is also a good method to investigate potential treatments for serious life-threatening conditions, as once again, by the time a traditional trial is completed, it may be found that many patients were denied life-saving treatment. Sequential analysis is also useful if there are ethical concerns about added risk of a new treatment.[26–28] In these cases, sequential analysis is a valid, cost-efficient approach used to detect a significant difference between groups as soon as possible.

As the outcome of each patient (or pair of patients) is established, a sequential line is plotted on a graph with preset boundary limits (Figure 4.5). If either of the two limits is broached, a conclusion of difference is made and the trial stopped (so, in effect, there is a statistical comparison made each time a preference is determined). If the boundary limits are not broached and the plotted line continues on to cross the right-hand boundary (the preset sample size limit), the trial is stopped and a conclusion of no difference is made. Boundary limits can be calculated for different significance levels (usually $P < 0.05$ or $P < 0.01$), using binomial probability (see Chapter 2) or a paired non-parametric test (see Chapters 5 and 6).

There are several other ways of developing and using boundary limits

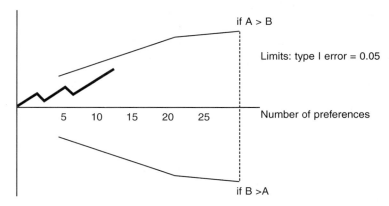

Figure 4.5 A sequential design comparing two treatments (A and B), using a *P* value of 0.05 as the stopping rule. A preference for A leads the line upwards and to the right; a preference for B leads the line downwards and to the right. When a boundary limit is crossed, a conclusion of significant difference is made

in sequential analysis. Some examples can be found in the anaesthetic literature; these include investigation of anaesthetic drug thrombo-phlebitis,[31] treatment of postoperative nausea and vomiting,[32] and use of low molecular weight heparin to prevent deep venous thrombosis after hip surgery.[33]

The above method of sequential analysis is seldom used in current medical research (unfortunately, College and Board examiners persist in asking about it!). A more appropriate modification is **interim analysis**.

Interim analysis

Interim analysis is also a method of repeatedly comparing groups while a trial is still in progress. But, in contrast to sequential analysis, these are preplanned statistical comparisons between groups (usually) on a restricted number of specified occasions during the trial. This approach has become the most common method to use when there is a requirement to stop a trial early, once sufficient evidence of significant difference is obtained, without jeopardizing statistical validity. A significant difference is inferred if one of these comparisons results in a *P* value that is smaller than a pre-specified value and the trial is generally stopped. Thus, each pre-specified type I error can be described as a '**stopping rule**'. Most commonly, two to four comparisons are made (usually after a certain proportion of patients are enrolled). The number and timing of these comparisons should be determined before the trial is commenced.

Interim analysis is universally employed in large, multi-centred trials. In many cases the interim analyses are performed blind, independent of the investigators, by a **Data and Safety Monitoring Committee**.[26,27] This has the strengths of maintaining patient safety and optimizing trial efficiency.

Because of the 'multiple looks' at the data, there is an increased likelihood of finding a significant difference between groups purely by chance – the type I error is inflated. Therefore an adjustment is required to each incremental P value accepted as significant in order to preserve the overall chosen type I error (usually set at 0.01 or 0.05). Most commonly, extreme P values (say $P < 0.0005$) are required to stop a trial in its early stages (when sample numbers are small), aiming to preserve most of the type I error for the later analyses.[25,27–30]

There are a number of recommended methods used to divide up the type I error in trials that incorporate interim analysis. These include the O'Brien–Fleming method, the Peto method and the Pocock method.[25,27–30] The O'Brien–Fleming method unevenly apportions the total type I error according to how many looks at the data are planned.[26,29,30] For example, a trial that is to have four interim analyses can have stopping rules of $P < 0.00001$, $P < 0.0012$, $P < 0.0077$ and $P < 0.017$, leaving a final P value < 0.024 (for an overall significance level of $P < 0.05$).

Examples from the cardiology literature are discussed in an excellent review from the Task Force of the Working Group on Arrhythmias of the European Society of Cardiology.[28]

Data accuracy and data checking

Accurate data collection is vital for valid conclusions to be made from research. Inaccuracies can be reduced by appropriate validation, calibration and operation of the measuring instrument. Accuracy is also threatened by errors in data recording and computer data entry. **Data entry** errors can be reduced by using computer scanning technology or dual data entry (with cross-checking). Unintended loss of data accuracy can occur due to **digit preference**, where the observer rounds off the measurement (most commonly to 0 or 5, or an even number). The observer may also simply round off the measurement to a level whereby precision is lost: this should not occur until the reporting stage, after completion of data entry and statistical processing. Conversely, data should not be reported to a greater level of precision than justified by the accuracy of the measuring instrument. Such fanciful precision reduces the paper's readability and, more importantly, its scientific credibility.

Before data are analysed, they should undergo a process of data checking and this often results in detection and correction of data entry errors. Reliable data entry can be optimized by restricting the values that can be entered onto a computer data base, by visual inspection of the resultant data file, or by logical checks of data output (range, **outliers**, or extreme degree of data spread). These procedures should not be overlooked, as they are nearly always productive and will ultimately save time by avoiding the reworking of the analyses and presentation of results.

Extreme values, or outliers, may be accurate and their inclusion can be problematic. There are five possible approaches:

1. Confirm data accuracy (and correct if necessary)
2. Exclude outliers in order to 'smooth' data distribution
3. Report different results with data included, and excluded (does this change the results – is it stable?)
4. Transform the data to 'smooth' the distribution (e.g. **log transformation**)
5. Study more patients in order to dilute the effect of the outliers.

Missing data

The handling of missing data in a research study is a contentious issue, with no hard and fast rules. It occurs most commonly in critical care specialties because of some valid clinical problem overriding the researcher's interests, equipment unavailability or malfunction. Ideally, the steps to be taken when there are missing data should be pre-determined during the planning stages of a research project in order to maintain reliable results. In most situations it is best to report the missing data and the reasons why they were missing, and then exclude such patients from the analyses. Care must be taken when doing this as it may redefine the study population, such that patients with missing data differ from those with complete data, and the final population may not represent that intended.

If it can be shown that the missing data occurred *randomly*, that is, there was no systematic difference (for all important characteristics) between the patients with complete data and those with missing data, then it may be acceptable to include the patients in the analyses.

It is sometimes reasonable to replace the missing value with an estimate (usually derived from the group average), or if there are measurements of the variable at other time points, then using an average of those values. For example, if there is a missing value for cardiac output at ICU admission in a group of 45 patients (i.e. 44 patients had complete data), and the group had an average cardiac output of 5.6 l/min at that time, it would be reasonable to record the value 5.6 for the individual with missing data. Alternatively, if the individual had a cardiac output recording of 4.8 l/min one hour earlier, and 5.2 l/min two hours later, then it may be appropriate to use an average of those two values (i.e. 5.0 l/min). Another approach is to use the 'carry-over rule', where the preceding measurement is used to replace the missing value. Each of these methods has its critics and is no substitute for accurate, complete data. The method chosen should be decided during the planning phase of the study and defined in the protocol, and not after data has been collected. Further discussion of this issue can be found elsewhere.[34,35]

Intention to treat

There are many reasons why patients may withdraw from a study or be lost to follow-up. They may also refuse the allocated treatment, unintentionally receive the comparator treatment, or receive other treatments which may affect the outcome of interest. Some investigators (and clinicians) only analyse those patients who received the study treatment (**per protocol analysis**). This approach seems intuitively obvious to many clinicians, as they are only interested in the effect of the actual treatment (not what happened to those who did not receive it). But a per protocol analysis can be misleading, particularly if the allocated treatment has side-effects or is ineffective in some patients. Per protocol analysis may then over-estimate the true benefit and under-estimate adverse effects. The most valid method is to use **intention to treat** analysis, so that all patients who were enrolled and randomly allocated to treatment are included in the analysis. This gives a more reliable estimate of true effect in routine practice because it replicates what we actually do – we consider a treatment and want to know what is most likely going to happen (thus accommodating for treatment failure, non-compliance, additional treatments, and so on).

Thus, if 20% of epidurals are ineffective, say because of failed insertion, displacement or inadequate management,[36] and a theoretical study demonstrates a reduction in major complications on per protocol analysis, it may be explained by an actual shift in group identity (Table 4.2). A real example can be found in the recent anaesthetic literature, where Bode *et al.*[37] found no significant effect of regional anaesthesia in peripheral vascular surgery on intention to treat analysis, but that those who had a failed regional technique had a higher mortality than those who did not.

A per protocol analysis is sometimes used appropriately when analysing adverse events in drug trials, as it can be argued that the side-effects of the actual treatment received is clinically relevant in that circumstance.

Table 4.2 Effect of how groups are analysed if four patients did not receive their allocated (epidural) treatment and were treated with patient-controlled anaesthesia (PCA) (and three of these had major complications). A per protocol analysis would consider these patients in the PCA group. The recommended approach is to use intention to treat analysis. The resultant *P* value of 0.33 suggests that the observed difference could be explained by chance

A. Per protocol analysis

	Epidural group (n = 16)	*PCA group* (n = 24)	*P value*
Complications	3 (19%)	13 (54%)	0.047

B. Intention to treat analysis

	Epidural group (n = 20)	*PCA group* (n = 20)	*P value*
Complications	6 (30%)	10 (50%)	0.33

References

1. Sackett DL. Bias in analytic research. J Chron Dis 1979; **32**:51–63.
2. Rothman KJ. Epidemiological methods in clinical trials. *Cancer* 1977; **39**:1771–1779.
3. Horwitz RI, Feinstein AR. Methodologic standards and contradictory results in case-control research. *Am J Med* 1979; **66**:556–562.
4. Rebollo MH, Bernal JM, Llorca J *et al.* Nosocomial infections in patients having cardiovascular operations: a multivariate analysis of risk factors. *J Thorac Cardiovasc Surg* 1996; **112**:908–913.
5. Sackett DL, Haynes RB, Guyatt GH *et al.* Clinical Epidemiology: A Basic Science for Clinical Medicine, 2nd ed. Boston: Little Brown, 1991:283–302.
6. Kurz A, Sessler DI, Lenhardt R. Perioperative normothermia to reduce the incidence of surgical wound infection and shorten hospitalization. *N Engl J Med* 1996; **334**:1209–1215.
7. Morris JA, Gardner MJ. Calculating confidence intervals for relative risks, odds ratios, and standardised ratios and rates. In: Gardner MJ, Altman DG. Statistics with Confidence – Confidence Intervals and Statistical Guidelines. London: *British Medical Journal*, 1989:50–63.
8. Myles PS, Olenikov I, Bujor MA *et al.* ACE-inhibitors, calcium antagonists and low systemic vascular resistance following cardiopulmonary bypass. A case-control study. *Med J Aust* 1993; **158**:675–677.
9. Strom BL, Berlin JA, Kinman JL *et al.* Parenteral ketorolac and risk of gastrointestinal and operative site bleeding. A postmarketing surveillance study. *JAMA* 1996; **275**:376–382.
10. Hill AB. The environment and disease: association or causation? *Proc Roy Soc Med* 1965:295–300.
11. Myles PS, Power I. Does ketorolac cause renal failure – how do we assess the evidence? *Br J Anaesth* 1998; **80**:420–421 [editorial].
12. Suen TKL, Gin T, Chen PP *et al.* Ondansetron 4 mg for the prevention of nausea and vomiting after minor laparoscopic gynaecological surgery. *Anaesth Intensive Care* 1994; **22**:142–146.
13. Fujii Y, Saitoh Y, Tanaka H *et al.* Prophylactic oral antiemetics for preventing postoperative nausea and vomiting: granisetron versus domperidone. *Anesth Analg* 1998; **87**:1404–1407.
14. Loius TA, Lavori PW, Bailar JC *et al.* Crossover and self-controlled designs in clinical research. *N Engl J Med* 1984; **310**:24–31.
15. Woods JR, Williams JG, Tavel M. The two-period crossover design in medical research. *Ann Intern Med* 1989; **110**:560–566.
16. Ngan Kee WD, Lam KK, Chen PP, Gin T. Comparison of patient-controlled epidural analgesia with patient-controlled intravenous analgesia using pethidine or fentanyl. *Anaesth Intensive Care* 1997; **25**:126–132.
17. Myles PS, Leong CK, Weeks AM *et al.* Early hemodynamic effects of left atrial administration of epinephrine after cardiac transplantation. *Anesth Analg* 1997; **84**:976–981.
18. Guyatt GH, Keller JL, Jaeschke R *et al.* The *n*-of-1 randomized controlled trial: clinical usefulness. Our three year experience. *Ann Intern Med* 1990; **112**:293–299.
19. Altman DG. Comparability of randomised groups. *Statistician* 1985; **34**:125–136.
20. Altman DG, Dore CJ. Randomisation and baseline comparisons in clinical trials. *Lancet* 1990; **335**:149–153.
21. Lavori PW, Louis TA, Bailar JC *et al.* Designs for experiments – parallel comparisons of treatment. *N Engl J Med* 1983; **309**:1291–1299.

22. Berry CB, Butler PJ, Myles PS. Lung management during cardiopulmonary bypass: is continuous positive airways pressure beneficial? *Br J Anaesth* 1993; **71**:864–868.
23. Armitage P. Statistical Methods in Medical Research. London: Blackwell Scientific Publications, 1985:239–245.
24. Treasure T, Macrae KD. Minimisation: the platinum standard for trials? *BMJ* 1998; **317**:362–363.
25. McPherson K. Statistics: the problem of examining accumulating data more than once. *N Engl J Med* 1974; **290**:501–502.
26. Armitage P. Sequential methods in clinical trials. *Am J Pub Health* 1958; **48**:1395–1402.
27. Pocock SJ. Statistical and ethical issues in monitoring clinical trials. *Stat Med* 1993; **12**:1459–1469.
28. Task Force of the Working Group on Arrhythmias of the European Society of Cardiology. The early termination of clinical trials: causes, consequences, and control – with special reference to trials in the field of arrhythmias and sudden death. *Circulation* 1994; **89**:2892–2907.
29. Geller NL, Pocock SJ. Interim analyses in randomized clinical trials: ramifications and guidelines for practitioners. *Biometrics* 1987; **43**:213–223.
30. O'Brien PC, Fleming TR. A multiple testing procedure for clinical trials. *Biometrics* 1979; **35**:549–556.
31. Boon J, Beemer GH, Bainbridge DJ *et al.* Postinfusion thrombophlebitis: effect of intravenous drugs used in anaesthesia. *Anaesth Intensive Care* 1981; **9**:23–27.
32. Abramowitz MD, Oh TH, Epstein BS *et al.* The antiemetic effect of droperidol following outpatient strabismus surgery in children. *Anesthesiology* 1983; **59**:579–583.
33. Samama CM, Clergue F, Barre J *et al.* Low molecular weight heparin associated with spinal anaesthesia and gradual compression stockings in total hip replacement surgery. *Br J Anaesth* 1997; **78**:660–665.
34. Shearer PR. Missing data in quantitative designs. *J Royal Statist Soc Ser C Appl Statist* 1973; **22**:135–140.
35. Ludington E, Dexter F. Statistical analysis of total labor pain using the visual analog scale and application to studies of analgesic effectiveness during childbirth. *Anesth Analg* 1998; **87**:723–727.
36. Burstal R, Hayes C, Lantry G *et al.* Epidural analgesia – a prospective audit of 1062 patients. *Anaesth Intensive Care* 1998; **26**:165–173.
37. Bode RH Jr, Lewis KP, Zarich SW *et al.* Cardiac outcome after peripheral vascular surgery. Comparison of general and regional anesthesia. *Anesthesiology* 1996; **84**:3–13.

5

Comparing groups: numerical data

Parametric tests	Non-parametric tests
–Student's *t*-test	–Mann–Whitney U test (Wilcoxon rank sum test)
–analysis of variance (ANOVA)	–Wilcoxon signed ranks test
–repeated measures ANOVA	–Kruskal–Wallis ANOVA
	–Friedman two-way ANOVA

Key points
- Numerical data that are normally distributed can be analysed with parametric tests.
- Student's *t*-test is a parametric test used to compare the means of two groups.
- The unpaired *t*-test is used to compare two dependent groups.
- A one-tailed *t*-test is used to look for a difference between two groups in only one direction (i.e. larger or smaller).
- Analysis of variance (ANOVA) is a parametric test used to compare the means of two or more groups.
- Mann–Whitney U test is a non-parametric equivalent to the unpaired *t*-test.
- Kruskal–Wallis test is a non-parametric equivalent of ANOVA.

Numerical data may be continuous or ordinal (see Chapter 1). Continuous data are sometimes further divided into ratio or interval scales, but this division does not influence the choice of statistical test. This chapter is concerned with the various methods used to compare the central tendency of two or more groups when the data are on a numerical scale.

Numerical data that are normally distributed can be analysed with parametric tests. These tests are based on the parameters that define a normal distribution: mean and standard deviation (or variance).

Parametric tests

The parametric tests assume that:

1. Data are on a numerical scale
2. The distribution of the underlying population is normal
3. The samples have the same variance ('**homogeneity of variances**')
4. Observations within a group are independent
5. The samples are randomly drawn from the population

If it is uncertain whether the data are normally distributed they can be plotted and visually inspected, and/or tested for normality, using one of a number of **goodness of fit** tests. One example is the **Kolmogorov–Smirnov test**.[1] This compares the sample data with a normal distribution and derives a *P* value; if *P* > 0.05 the null hypothesis is accepted (i.e. the sample data are not different from the normal distribution) and the data are considered to be normally distributed.

Non-normal, or skewed, data can be transformed so that they approximate a normal distribution.[2–4] The commonest method is a **log transformation**, whereby the natural logarithms of the raw data are analysed to calculate a mean and standard deviation. The antilogarithm of the mean of this transformed data is known as the **geometric mean**. If the transformed data are shown to approximate a normal distribution, they can then be analysed with parametric tests.

Large sample (studies with, say, *n* > 100) data approximate a normal distribution and can nearly always be analysed with parametric tests.

The requirement for observations within a group to be independent means that multiple measurements from the same subject cannot be treated as separate individual observations. Thus, if three measurements are made on each of 12 subjects, these data cannot be considered as 36 independent samples. This is a special case of **repeated measures** and requires specific analyses (see later). The requirement for samples to be drawn randomly from a population is rarely achieved in clinical trials,[5] but this is not considered to be a major problem as results from inferential statistical tests have proved to be reliable in circumstances where this rule was not followed.

Student's t-test

Student's *t*-test is used to test the null hypothesis that there is no difference between two means. It is used in three circumstances:

- to test if a sample mean (as an estimate of a population mean) differs significantly from a given population mean (this is a **one-sample *t*-test**)
- to test if the population means estimated by two independent samples differ significantly (the **unpaired *t*-test**)
- to test if the population means estimated by two dependent samples differ significantly (the **paired *t*-test**).

The *t*-test can be used when the underlying assumptions of parametric tests are satisfied (see above). However the *t*-test is considered to be a robust test, in that it can accommodate some deviation from these assumptions. This is one of the reasons why it has been a popular test in clinical trials, where small samples (say *n* < 30) are commonly studied.

The *t*-test only compares the means of the two groups. Without formally testing the assumption of equal variance, it is possible to accept the null hypothesis and conclude that the samples come from the same population when they in fact come from two different populations that have similar means but different variances. The group variances can be compared using the F **test**. The F test is the ratio of variances (var_1/var_2);

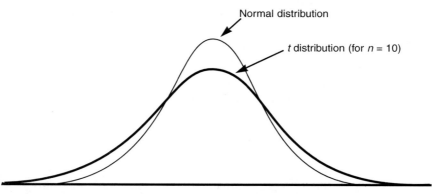

Figure 5.1 How a t distribution (for $n = 10$) compares with a normal distribution. A t distribution is broader and flatter, such that 95% of observations lie within the range mean $\pm t \times$ SD ($t = 2.23$ for $n = 10$) compared with mean ± 1.96 SD for the normal distribution

if F differs significantly from 1.0 then it is concluded that the group variances differ significantly.*

The t distribution was calculated by W.L. Gosset of the Guinness Brewing Company under the pseudonym Student (company policy prevented him from using his real name). A sample from a population with a normal distribution is also normally distributed if the sample size is large. With smaller sample sizes, the likelihood of extreme values is greater, so the distribution 'curve' is flatter and broader (Figure 5.1). The t distribution, like the normal distribution, is also bell shaped, but has wider dispersion – this accommodates for the unreliability of the sample standard deviation as an estimate of the population standard deviation.

There is a t distribution curve for any particular sample size and this is identified by denoting the t distribution at a given **degree of freedom**. Degrees of freedom is equal to one less than the sample size (d.f. $= n - 1$). It describes the number of independent observations available. As the degrees of freedom increases, the t distribution approaches the normal distribution. Thus, if you refer to a t-table in a reference text you can see that, as the degrees of freedom increases, the value of t approaches 1.96 at a P value of 0.05. This is analogous to a normal distribution where 5% of values lie outside 1.96 standard deviations from the mean.

The t-test is mostly used for small samples. When the sample size is large (say, $n > 100$), the sampling distribution is nearly normal and it is possible to use a test based on the normal distribution (z test). Theoretically, the t-test can be used even if the sample sizes are very small ($n < 10$), as long as the variables are normally distributed within each group and the variation of scores in the two groups is not too different.

*The value of F that defines a significant difference (say $P < 0.05$) depends on the sample size (degrees of freedom); this can be found in reference tables (F table) or can be calculated using statistical software.

The simplified formulae for the different forms of the *t*-test are:

1. One-sample t-test

$$t = \frac{\bar{X} - \mu}{\text{SE}}$$

where $\bar{X}$ = sample mean, μ = population mean, and SE = standard error.

2. Unpaired t-test

$$t = \frac{\bar{X}_1 - \bar{X}_2}{\text{SE}_{\bar{X}_1 - \bar{X}_2}}$$

where $\bar{X}_1 - \bar{X}_2$ is the difference between the means of the two groups, and SE denotes the standard error of this difference.*

3. Paired t-test

$$t = \frac{\bar{d}}{\text{SE}_{\bar{d}}}$$

where $\bar{d}$ is the mean difference, and SE denotes the standard error of this difference.

In each of these cases a P value can be obtained from a *t*-table in a reference text. More commonly now, a P value is derived using statistical software. The P value quantifies the likelihood of the observed difference occurring by chance alone. The null hypothesis (no difference) is rejected if the P value is less than the chosen **type I error** (α). Thus, it can be concluded that the sample(s) are subsets of different populations.

The t value can also be used to derive **95% confidence intervals** (95% CI).[7] In Chapter 3 we described how 95% CI can be calculated as the mean $\pm$ (1.96 $\times$ standard error). In small samples it is preferable to use the value of t rather than 1.96:

1. 95% CI of the group mean = mean $\pm$ (t value $\times$ SE)
2. 95% CI of the difference between groups = mean difference $\pm$ (t value $\times$ SE of the difference).

If the 95% CI of the difference between groups does not include zero (i.e. no difference), then there is a significant difference between groups at the 0.05 level. Thus, the 95% CI gives an estimate of precision, as well as indirectly giving the information about the probability of the observed difference being due to chance.

For example, Scheinkestel *et al.*[8] studied the effect of hyperbaric oxygen (HBO) therapy in patients with carbon monoxide poisoning. They reported the following results for a verbal learning test (with higher scores indicating better function): HBO group 42 vs. control (normal

---

*The SE is calculated from a pooled standard deviation that is a weighted average of the two sample variances:

$$\text{SE} = \sqrt{\frac{\text{Var}_1(n_1 - 1) + \text{Var}_2(n_2 - 1)}{n_1 + n_2 - 2}} \cdot \sqrt{\frac{1}{n_1} + \frac{1}{n_2}}$$

oxygen) group 49.2. The mean difference was –7.2 and the 95% CI of the difference was –12.2 to –2.2. Thus, the 95% CI did not include the zero value, and so it can be concluded that there was a statistically significant difference between groups. The interval 2.2–12.2 was fairly wide and so the study did not have high precision for this estimate of effect. The authors concluded that HBO therapy does not improve outcome in carbon monoxide poisoning.

Unpaired vs. paired tests

Unpaired tests are used when two different ('independent') groups are compared. Paired tests are used when the two samples are matched or paired ('dependent'): the usual setting is when measurements are made on the same subjects before and after a treatment.

It is useful to try and reduce variability within the sample group to make more apparent the difference between groups. In the *t*-test, this has the effect of reducing the denominator and making the *t* value larger. With all samples, there is variability of inherent characteristics that may influence the variable under study. For example, in a two-group unpaired comparison of a drug to lower blood pressure, different patients will have a variety of factors that may affect the blood pressure immediately before intervention. These initial differences contribute to the total variability within each group (**variance**). By using the same subjects twice in a *before and after treatment* design, there is reduced individual and total within group variance.

Another example of a paired design is a crossover design of two treatments when instead of using two groups, each receiving one treatment, the same group receives the two drugs on two separate occasions (see Chapter 4). Because the same group of patients is used, there is less variability.

In the analysis of paired designs, instead of treating each group separately and analysing raw scores, we can look only at the *differences* between the two measures in each subject. By subtracting the first score from the second for each subject and then analysing only those differences, we will exclude the variation in our data set that results from unequal baseline levels of individual subjects. Thus a smaller sample size can be used in a paired design to achieve the same **power** as an unpaired design.

It is useful to take another view of the *t*-test procedure because it may be helpful in understanding the basis of **analysis of variance**. When comparing central location between samples, we actually compare the difference (or variability) *between* samples with the variability *within* samples. Intuitively, if the variability between sample means is very large and the variability within a sample is very low, then it will be easier to detect a difference between the means. Conversely if the difference between means is very small and the variability within the sample is very large, it will become more difficult to detect a difference.

If we look at the formula for the *t*-test, the difference between means is the numerator. If this is small relative to the variance within the samples (the denominator), the resultant t value will be small and we are less likely to reject the null hypothesis (Figure 5.2).

(a)

(b)

(c)

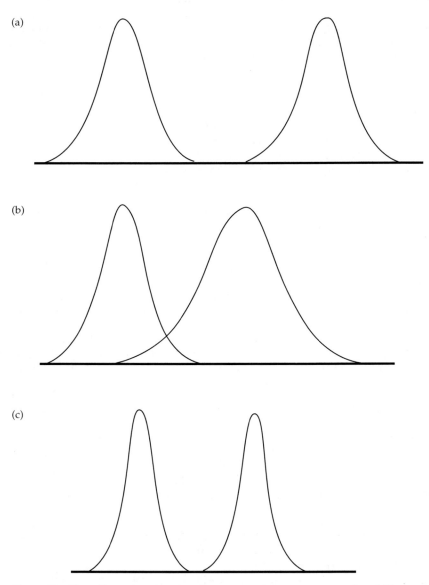

Figure 5.2 The effect of variance: when comparing two groups, the ability to detect a difference between group means is affected by not only the absolute difference but also the group variance. (a) Two curves of sampling distributions with no overlap and easily detected difference; (b) means now closer together causing overlap of curves and possibility of not detecting a difference; (c) means same distance as in B but smaller variance so that there is no overlap and difference easy to detect

If there is reason to look for a difference between mean values in only one direction (i.e. larger or smaller), then a **one-tailed *t*-test** can be used. This essentially doubles the chance of finding a significant difference (i.e. increases power) (Figure 5.3). Some investigators have used a one-tailed *t*-test because a two-tailed test failed to show a significant ($P < 0.05$) result. This should not be done. A one-tailed *t*-test should only be used if there is a valid reason for investigating a difference in only one direction.[9] Ideally this should be based on known effects of the treatment and be outlined in the study protocol before results are analysed (**a priori**).

Comparing more than two groups

The *t*-test should not be used to compare three or more groups.[10,11] Although it is possible to divide three groups into three different pairs and use the *t*-test for each pair, this will increase the chance of making a type I error (conducting three *t* tests will have approximately a 3α-fold chance of making a type I error).

If we consider a seven-group study, there are 21 possible pairs and an α of 0.05, or 1/20 for each would make it likely that one of the observed differences could have easily occurred by chance. The probability of getting at least one significant result is $1–0.95^{21} = 0.66$. There is a better way to conduct **multiple comparisons**.

It is possible to divide the α value for each test by the number of comparisons so that overall, the type I error is limited to the original α.[1] For example, if there are three *t*-tests, then an α of 0.05 would be reduced to 0.0167 for each test and only if the *P* value was less than this adjusted α would we reject the null hypothesis. This maintains a probability of 0.05 of making a type I error overall. This is known as the **Bonferroni correction**.

However, it is apparent that as the number of comparisons increases, the adjusted α becomes so small that it could be very unlikely to find a

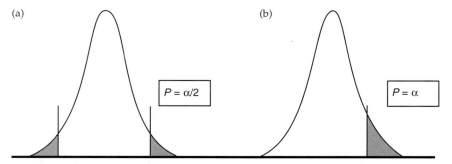

Figure 5.3 Two-tailed and one-tailed *t*-tests. A one-tailed *t*-test is used to look for a difference between mean values in only one direction (i.e. larger or smaller). This increases the likelihood of showing a significant difference (power). (a) For two-tailed α = 0.05, and a normal distribution the critical *z* value is 1.96; (b) for one-tailed α = 0.05, and a normal distribution, the critical *z* value is 1.645

difference and we risk making more type II errors. Thus the Bonferroni correction is a conservative approach. The best way to avoid this is to limit the number of comparisons.

The comparison of means from multiple groups is better carried out using a family of techniques broadly known as **analysis of variance** (**ANOVA**).[6,11] Thus one important reason for using ANOVA methods rather than multiple *t*-tests is that ANOVA is more powerful (i.e. more efficient at detecting a true difference).

Analysis of variance (ANOVA)

In general, the purpose of ANOVA is to test for significant differences between the means of two or more groups.[6] It seems contradictory that a test that compares means is actually called analysis of variance. However, to determine differences between means, we are actually comparing the ratio of two variances – ANOVA is based on the **F test** of variance.

From our discussion of the *t*-test, a significant result was more likely when the difference between means is much greater than the variance within the samples. With ANOVA, we also compare the difference between the means (using variance as our measure of dispersion) with the variance within the samples. The test first asks if the difference between groups can be explained by the degree of spread (variance) within a group. It divides up the total variability (variance) into the variance *within* each group, and that *between* each group. If the observed variance between groups is greater than that within groups, then there is a significant difference.

These two variances are sometimes known as the between-group variability and within-group variability. The within-group variability is also known as the error variance because it is variation that we cannot readily account for in the study design, being based on random differences in our samples. However we hope that the between-group, or effect variance, is the result of our treatment. We can compare these two estimates of variance using the F test.

There are many types of ANOVA and the only two we will consider here are the extensions of the unpaired and paired *t*-test to circumstances where there are more than two groups. Like the *t*-test, ANOVA uses the same assumptions that apply to parametric tests. A simplified formula for the F statistic is:

$$F = \frac{MS_b}{MS_w}$$

where MS is the mean squares between and within groups.

The formulae for mean squares are complex. If k represents the number of groups and N the total number of results for all groups, the variation between groups has degrees of freedom $k-1$, and the variation within groups has degrees of freedom $N-k$. Thus if one uses reference tables to look at critical value of the F distribution, the two degrees of freedom must be used to locate the correct entry.

If only two means are compared, ANOVA will give the same results as the *t*-test.* In an analogous manner to the *t*-test described earlier, the F statistic calculated from the samples is compared with known values of the F distribution. A large F value indicates that it is more unlikely that the null hypothesis is true. Decisions on accepting or rejecting the null hypothesis are based on preset choices for α, the chosen type I error.

If we simply compare the means of three or more groups, the ANOVA is often referred to as a one-way or one-factor ANOVA. There is also two-way ANOVA when two grouping factors are analysed, and multiple analysis of variance (**MANOVA**) when multiple grouping factors are analysed. Another method is the **general linear model** (GLM), a form of **multivariate regression**. The GLM calculates R^2, a measure of effect size. R^2 is mathematically related to F and *t*.

An example of one-way ANOVA would be to compare the changes in blood pressure after the administration of three different drugs. One may then consider additional contributory factors by looking at, for example, a gender-based difference in effect. This would be a two-factor (drug treatment and gender) ANOVA. In such a case the ANOVA will return a *P* value for the difference based on drug treatment and another *P* value for the difference based on gender. There will also be a *P* value for the **interaction** of drug treatment and gender, indicating perhaps, for example, that one drug treatment may be more likely to cause an effect in female patients.

ANOVA is a **multivariate** statistical technique because it can test each factor while controlling for all other factors and also enable us to detect interaction effects between variables. Thus more complex hypotheses can be tested and this is another reason why ANOVA is more powerful than using multiple *t*-tests.

However, if the ANOVA returns a significant result, the ANOVA by itself will only tell us that there is a difference, not where the difference lies. So if we are comparing three samples, a significant result will not identify which sample mean is different to any other. Clearly this is not that useful and we must make use of further tests (*post hoc* **tests**) to identify the differences.[6]

One confusing aspect of ANOVA is that there are many *post hoc* tests and there is not universal agreement among statisticians as to which tests are preferred.[6] Statistical software packages often provide a limited selection. Of the common tests, the **Fisher Protected Least Significant Difference (LSD)** is the least conservative (i.e. most likely to indicate significant differences) and the **Scheffé test** is the most conservative but the most versatile because it can test complex hypotheses involving combinations of group means. For comparisons of specifically selected pairs of means, tests such as **Tukey's Honestly Significant Difference (HSD)** and **Newman–Keuls** are often used. **Dunnett's test** is used specifically when one wishes to test just one sample mean against all the others.

---

*Numerically $F = t^2$.

Repeated measures ANOVA

As an extension of the paired *t*-test, we can imagine situations where we take repeated measurements of the same variable under different conditions or at different points in time. It is very common to have repeated measures designs in anaesthesia, but the analysis of these is complex and fraught with hazard.[11]

An example is a study by Myles *et al.*,[12] who measured quality of recovery scores on each of three days after surgery in four groups of patients (Figure 5.4). They found a reduction in quality of recovery scores early after surgery in all groups, followed by a gradual improvement. There were no significant differences between groups with ANOVA and so *post hoc* tests looking at each time interval were not performed.

Although repeated measures designs can be very useful in analysing this type of data, some of the assumptions of ANOVA may not be met and this casts doubt on the validity of the analysis.[11] **Homogeneity of variance** can be a problem because there is usually greater variation at very low readings (assays at the limit of detection) or very high readings. Transformation of data can be a possible solution.[2] A more important consideration is analysis of **residuals**. Here the difference between the group mean and individual values ('residuals') are analysed to check that they are normally distributed.

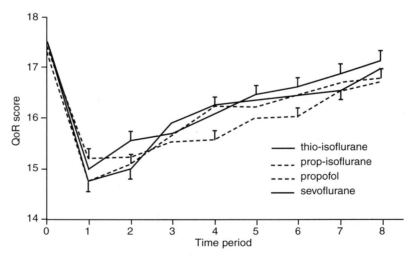

Figure 5.4 Perioperative changes in mean quality of recovery (QoR) score (after Myles *et al.*[12]). From this graph, one can easily imagine all the possible comparisons that one could make between different points on the curves, with the attendant problems of multiple comparisons. Time periods
0 = preoperative, 1 = recovery room discharge, 2 = at 2–4 h postoperatively, 3 = day 1 (am), 4 = day 1 (pm), 5 = day 2 (am), 6 = day 2 (pm), 7 = day 3 (am), 8 = day 3 (pm)

One of the assumptions of repeated measures ANOVA is compound symmetry, also known as **multisample sphericity**. This means that the outcome data should not only have the same variance at each time but also that the correlations between all pairs of repeated measurements in the same subject are equal. This is not usually the case. In the typical repeated measures examples above, values at adjacent dose or time points are likely to be closer to one another than those further apart. If uncorrected, the risk of type I error is increased. Correction factors include the **Greenhouse–Geisser** and **Hunyh–Feldt**.[11]

It is often possible to simplify the data and use summary measures of the important features of each curve to compare the groups.[13] A simple unpaired *t*-test can then be used to compare these summary measures between groups. Some measures include:[13]

- time to peak effect
- area under a time–response curve
- mean effect over time.

For example, drug absorption profiles are conventionally summarized by three results: (a) the time to peak concentration (t_{max}), (b) the actual peak concentration (C_{max}), (c) the area under the curve (AUC) to a certain time point as a measure of overall absorption. In a comparison of the interpleural injection of bupivacaine with and without adrenaline,[14] a Mann–Whitney U test was used to show that t_{max} was delayed and C_{max} was decreased in the adrenaline group (Figure 5.5). The conclusion was

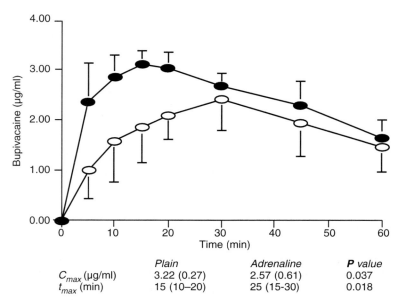

	Plain	Adrenaline	**P** value
C_{max} (µg/ml)	3.22 (0.27)	2.57 (0.61)	0.037
t_{max} (min)	15 (10–20)	25 (15-30)	0.018

Figure 5.5 Absorption of bupivacaine after interpleural administration with (empty symbols) and without (plain, full symbols) adrenaline. The addition of adrenaline delays systemic absorption of bupivacaine.[14] Mean (SD) and median (range) pharmacokinetic data are detailed below

that the addition of adrenaline did decrease systemic absorption of bupivacaine.

As another example, when paracetamol was used as a measure of gastric emptying in intensive care patients,[15] the AUC to 30 min was less in patients with intracranial hypertension, indicating delayed emptying when compared with patients without intracranial hypertension.

As a more complex example, we may want to compare the haemo-dynamic stability of two induction agents in a special patient group. We might inject the drug and measure systolic arterial pressure for the first 5 min after injection. For each drug we might want to know: (a) the time to maximum effect, and (b) the greatest change from baseline. These would be analogous to the t_{max} and C_{max} in the previous example. However we may also want to know: (a) when the blood pressure first changes from the baseline (latency), (b) when the blood pressure returns to normal, and (c) whether or not these variables are different for each drug.

Rather than conduct multiple paired t-tests against the baseline blood pressure, a repeated measures ANOVA is more appropriate. Note that within each group, one can perform a repeated measures ANOVA to compare the baseline data with subsequent readings. To test whether or not there are any differences between groups, one would conduct a repeated measures ANOVA on both groups at the same time, using group as a factor. One can see that ANOVA designs can become quite complex.

Note that these patients will have different baseline blood pressures. Repeated measures ANOVA will take into account the different baseline blood pressures when comparing subsequent differences. However, if the baseline blood pressure is quite variable, then absolute changes may be slightly misleading. A drop in blood pressure of 30 mmHg is probably more significant in someone with a baseline of 100 mmHg than one with a baseline of 150 mmHg. This has led some authors to convert absolute differences into percentage changes from baseline before analysis.

Another question may be to determine if, overall, there is a greater change in blood pressure in one group than the other. This can pose further problems. In a manner similar to the AUC for the drug absorption examples, one could calculate the AUC or other summary measures such as the mean or sum of the blood pressure readings in each patient. However if the time limit chosen is too long, one may not detect any differences between groups because the blood pressure has long returned to normal and this would obscure any initial differences. It is not appropriate to recalculate the summary measure at every time point to find significant differences ('data dredging').

The ANOVA and summary measures can also obscure extreme data. We may have to make a clinical judgment on whether it is important to distinguish a rapid but short duration of severe hypotension in one group from a more sustained less severe drop in blood pressure in the other group. Similarly, we would be interested if one drug occasionally causes very severe hypotension.

From this discussion of a common and apparently simple question, one can see that there are many possible multiple comparisons that would inflate the type I error, even with ANOVA – and we have not even considered mean arterial pressure, heart rate and other cardiovascular variables! The investigator is well advised to precisely define the important hypotheses in advance (*a priori*) so that the appropriate selected analyses are undertaken.

A dose–response study of an analgesic presents similar problems. We may want to know the onset of action, maximal effect, duration and overall efficacy of each dose. If the primary measure is a pain visual analogue score (**VAS**), then non-parametric ANOVA tests may be more appropriate. In a dose–response study of epidural pethidine,[16] pain scores were measured at 3-minute intervals and the onset of action was defined as the time taken to decrease the initial pain score by 50%. This summary measure was then compared among groups using a Kruskal– Wallis test followed by Mann–Whitney U tests. Overall postoperative analgesia was also analysed by comparing the area under the curve of the pain VAS among the three groups. In both cases, a repeated measures analysis of the pain scores (to determine when the pain score was different from the baseline) could have been theoretically used but would have added complexity without any further useful clinical information. In both these studies, non-parametric tests were used to compare VAS measurements because these data were considered ordinal data. However, the use of parametric *t*-tests and ANOVA is considered acceptable (see Chapter 1).

ANOVA is a powerful statistical technique and many complex analyses are possible. However there are also many pitfalls, especially with repeated measures ANOVA. Advice and assistance from an experienced statistician is highly recommended. Other computer-intensive tests have also been advocated for comparing means.[5]

Non-parametric tests

When the assumptions for the parametric tests are not met, there are many non-parametric alternatives for the parametric tests described above.[1] These include:

1. Mann–Whitney U test (identical to the Wilcoxon rank sum) is a non-parametric equivalent to the unpaired Student's *t*-test
2. Wilcoxon signed ranks test is a non-parametric equivalent to the paired Student's *t*-test
3. Kruskal–Wallis test is a non-parametric equivalent of one-way ANOVA
4. Friedman's test is a non-parametric repeated measures ANOVA
5. Spearman rank order (rho) is a non-parametric version of the Pearson correlation coefficient *r* (see Chapter 7)

Many other non-parametric tests are available,[1] but these are not often used in anaesthesia research. Non-parametric tests do not assume a normal distribution and so are sometimes referred to as distribution-free tests. They are best used when small samples are selected because in these circumstances it is unlikely that the data can be demonstrated to be normally distributed.

Non-parametric tests do however have some underlying assumptions:

1. Data are from a continuous distribution of at least ordinal scale
2. Observations within a group are independent
3. Samples have been drawn randomly from the population

Non-parametric tests convert the raw results into ranks and then perform calculations on these ranks to obtain a test statistic. The calculations are generally easier to perform than for the parametric tests.

However, non-parametric tests may fail to detect a significant difference (which a parametric test may). That is, they usually have less **power**.

Just as described above for the parametric tests, the test statistic is compared with known values for the sampling distribution of that statistic and the null hypothesis is accepted or rejected. With these tests, the null hypothesis is that the samples come from populations with the same median.

Statistical programs may use approximations to determine the sampling distribution of the test statistic, especially when the sample size is large. For example, in the case of the Mann–Whitney U test, one approach has been to perform an unpaired *t*-test on the ranks (rather than the original raw scores) and, strictly speaking, this normal approximation actually compares the mean ranks of the data between two groups rather than the medians.

Mann–Whitney U test (Wilcoxon rank sum test)

This test is used to determine whether or not two independent groups have been drawn from the same population. It is a very useful test because it can have high power (≈ 0.95), compared with the unpaired *t*-test, even when all the conditions of the latter are satisfied.[1] It has fewer assumptions and can be more powerful than the *t*-test when conditions for the latter are not satisfied. The test has several names because Mann, Whitney and Wilcoxon all described tests that were essentially identical in analysis but presented them differently.

The Mann–Whitney U test is the recommended test to use when comparing two groups that have data measured on an ordinal scale.[17] However, if the data represent a variable that is, in effect, a continuous quantity, then a *t*-test may be used if the data are normally distributed. This is more likely with large samples (say, $n > 100$).[17]

In the Wilcoxon rank sum test, data from both the groups are combined and treated as one large group. Then the data are ordered and given ranks, separated back into their original groups, and the ranks in each group are then added to give the test statistic for each group. Tied data are given the same rank, calculated as the mean rank of the tied observations. The test then determines whether or not the sum of ranks in one group is different from that in the other. The sum of all the ranks is $N(N + 1)/2$, where N is the total number of observations.

For example, a hypothetical study investigating the effect of gender on postoperative headache may measure this pain on a 100 mm visual analogue scale. Each patient would have their pain score recorded and they would be ranked from lowest to highest (Table 5.1).

Wilcoxon signed ranks test

It is important to distinguish this test from the similar sounding unpaired test above. This is also a very valuable test with good efficiency (power

Table 5.1 A hypothetical study investigating the effect of gender on postoperative headache in 30 patients (16 male, 14 female). Pain is measured on a 100 mm visual analogue scale. Each patient has their pain score ranked from lowest to highest. Tied data are given the same rank, calculated as the mean rank of the tied observations

Patients	Male group Pain score	rank	Patients	Female group Pain score	rank
1	8	5	1	16	12
2	11	8	2	28	19.5
3	5	2	3	68	28
4	12	9	4	37	22
5	6	3.5	5	21	16
6	22	17	6	40	23
7	46	25	7	28	19.5
8	14	10	8	27	18
9	6	3.5	9	43	24
10	31	21	10	60	27
11	15	11	11	90	30
12	20	15	12	4	1
13	18	14	13	78	29
14	9	6	14	53	26
15	17	13			
16	10	7			
Sum of ranks	$W_1 = 170$			$W_2 = 295$	
Mean rank	$R_1 = 10.44$			$R_2 = 21.07$	
Standard deviation	6.67			7.79	

1. Exact method
Use the group sum of ranks and consult a reference table for group sizes 16 and 14. Because W_1 lies outside the quoted range (at $P < 0.05$), the null hypothesis can be rejected.

2. Normal approximation
The mean rank in the male group ($n = 16$) is 10.44, with a standard deviation of 6.67. The mean rank in the female group ($n = 14$) is 21.07, with a standard deviation of 7.79. The pooled standard deviation (see footnote on page 54) is 7.21. The degrees of freedom are 16 + 14 − 2 = 28. The t statistic based on ranks is:

$$t = \frac{\text{Difference between ranks}}{\text{SE of the rank difference}}$$

$$= \frac{21.07 - 10.44}{7.21 \sqrt{(1/16 + 1/14)}}$$

$$= \frac{10.63}{2.64}$$

$$= 4.03$$

⇒ 4.03 is greater than the t value (2.048) for d.f. = 28, so $P < 0.05$

$\approx 95\%$) compared with the paired t-test.[1] As in the paired t-test, the differences between pairs are calculated but then the absolute differences are ranked (without regard to whether they are positive or negative). The positive or negative signs of the original differences are preserved and assigned back to the corresponding ranks when calculating the test statistic. The sum of the positive ranks is compared with the sum of the negative ranks. If there is no difference between groups, we would expect the sum of the positive ranks to be equal to the sum of the negative ranks.

Kruskal–Wallis ANOVA

This tests the null hypothesis that k independent groups come from populations with the same median. A formula for the Kruskal–Wallis test statistic is:[1]

$$KW = \frac{12}{N(N + 1)} \sum_{j = 1}^{k} n_j (\bar{R}_j - \bar{R})^2$$

where N = the total number of cases, k = the number of groups, n_j = the number of cases in the jth sample, $\bar{R}_j$ = the average of the ranks in the jth group, and $\bar{R}$ = the average of all the ranks (and equal to $[N + 1]/2$).

If a significant difference is found, *post hoc* comparisons are usually performed with the Mann–Whitney U test with a **Bonferroni correction**. This approach does not consider all group data and a method based on group mean ranks can also be used.[1]

Friedman two-way ANOVA

This tests the null hypothesis that k repeated measures or matched groups come from populations with the same median. *Post hoc* tests need to be performed if a significant difference is found. These tests are unfortunately not available with most statistical software packages but can be found in specialized texts.[1]

References

1. Siegal S, Castellan NJ Jr. Non-parametric Statistics for the Behavioral Sciences 2nd ed. McGraw-Hill, New York 1988.
2. Bland JM, Altman DG. Transforming data. *Br Med J* 1996; **312**:770.
3. Bland JM, Altman DG. Transformations, means, and confidence intervals. *Br Med J* 1996; **312**: 1079.
4. Bland JM, Altman DG. The use of transformation when comparing two means. *Br Med J* 1996; **312**:1153.
5. Ludbrook J. Issues in biomedical statistics: comparing means by computer-intensive tests. *Aust NZ J Surg* 1995; **65**:812–819.
6. Godfrey K. Comparing the means of several groups. *N Engl J Med* 1985; **313**:1450–1456.
7. Gardner MJ, Altman DG. Statistics with Confidence – Confidence Intervals and Statistical Guidelines. *British Medical Journal*, London 1989:pp20–27.

8. Scheinkestel CD, Bailey M, Myles PS *et al.* Hyperbaric or normobaric oxygen for acute carbon monoxide poisoning – a randomized, controlled clinical trial. *Med J Aust* 1999; **170**:203–210.
9. Bland JM, Altman DG. One and two sided tests of significance. *Br Med J* 1994; **309**:248.
10. Bland JM, Altman DG. Multiple significance tests: the Bonferroni method. *Br Med J* 1995; **310**:170.
11. Ludbrook J. Repeated measurements and multiple comparisons in cardiovascular research. *Cardiovasc Res* 1994; **28**:303–311.
12. Myles PS, Hunt JO, Fletcher H *et al.* Propofol, thiopental, sevoflurane and isoflurane: a randomized controlled trial of effectiveness study. *Anesth Analg* in press.
13. Matthews JNS, Altman DG, Campbell MJ *et al.* Analysis of serial measurements in medical research. *BMJ* 1990; **300**:230–235.
14. Gin T, Chan K, Kan AF *et al.* Effect of adrenaline on venous plasma concentrations of bupivacaine after interpleural administration. *Br J Anaesth* 1990; **64**:662–666.
15. McArthur CJ, Gin T, McLaren IM *et al.* Gastric emptying following brain injury: effects of choice of sedation and intracranial pressure. *Intensive Care Med* 1995; **21**:573–576.
16. Ngan Kee WD, Lam KK, Chen PP, Gin T. Epidural meperidine after cesarean section: the effect of diluent volume. *Anesth Analg* 1997; **85**:380–384.
17. Moses LE, Emerson JD, Hosseini H. Analyzing data from ordered categories. *N Engl J Med* 1984; **311**:442–448.

6

Comparing groups: categorical data

Chi-square	**Risk ratio and odds ratio**
−Yates' correction	**Number needed to treat**
Fisher's exact test	**Mantel–Haenszel test**
The binomial test	**Kappa statistic**
McNemar's chi-square test	

Key points
- The chi-square test is used to compare independent groups of categorical data.
- Yates' correction factor should be used when the sample size is small.
- The results from two group comparisons with two categories are set out in a 2 × 2 contingency table.
- Fisher's exact test is a recommended alternative for analysing data from 2 × 2 tables.
- McNemar's test is used to compare paired groups of categorical data.
- The risk ratio is the proportion of patients with an outcome who were exposed to a risk factor vs. the proportion not exposed.
- Odds ratio is an estimate of risk ratio, used mostly in retrospective case-control studies.
- The number needed to treat (NNT) is the reciprocal of the absolute risk reduction.
- The kappa statistic is a measure of agreement.

Categorical data are nominal and can be counted (see Chapter 1). This chapter is concerned with various methods to compare two or more groups when the data are categorical. Extensive further reading is available in a textbook on non-parametric statistics by Siegal and Castellan.[1]

Chi-square (χ^2)

The **Pearson chi-square (χ^2) test** is the most common significance test used for comparing groups of categorical data. It compares frequencies and tests whether the observed rate differs significantly from that expected if there were no difference between groups (i.e. the **null hypothesis**).

The calculated value of the Pearson χ^2 test statistic is compared to the **chi-square distribution**, a continuous frequency distribution, and the resultant significance level (*P* value) depends on the overall number of observations and the number of cells in the table. The χ^2 distribution is derived from the square of standard normal variables (X) and provides a basis for calculating the *t* and F distributions described in the previous chapter. It consists of a family of curves, each of which, like the *t*-test, has

Table 6.1 A 2 × 2 contingency table

	Group A	Group B	Row total
Outcome 1	a	b	a + b
Outcome 2	c	d	c + d
Column total	a + c	b + d	a + b + c + d = N

its **degrees of freedom.*** The degrees of freedom describes the number of independent observations available, and for categorical data is determined by the number of cells in the contingency table (see later).

The χ^2 frequency distribution is a very important and fundamental distribution in statistics and its use is not just confined to the situations below. Confusion occurs because the Pearson χ^2 is often just called the χ^2 test and one might think that the χ^2 distribution is unique to the Pearson χ^2 statistic just as the t distribution is associated with the t statistic. Many test statistics apart from the Pearson χ^2 are referred to the χ^2 distribution.

The Pearson χ^2 test assumes that:

- the expected frequencies are not very small
- observations within a group are independent
- the samples are randomly drawn from the population

Note that this first assumption pertains to the *expected* frequency and not the *observed* frequency in the study. If the study sample is small (say, $n < 40$) and expected frequencies are low, then it may be more appropriate to use an **exact test** (i.e. a different method of analysis, see later). The requirement for observations within a group to be independent means that multiple counts from the same subject cannot be treated as separate individual observations. Thus, if three counts are made on each of 12 subjects, these data cannot be considered as 36 independent samples. This is **paired (dependent) data** and requires specific analyses (see later). The requirement for random selection of subjects from a defined population is rarely achieved in medical research but does not appear to be a major problem. The exact methods do not have this assumption.[2]

Let us first consider the most common situation where there are two independent groups and two mutually exclusive outcomes. Having only two possible outcomes means that in effect we are comparing **proportions** in the two groups. The data are summarized in a 2 × 2 **contingency table** of frequencies (Table 6.1).

The row totals and column totals are also called the marginal frequencies. Surprisingly, there are over 20 statistical tests that can be applied to 2 × 2 tables of this sort and the Pearson χ^2, although the most commonly used, is not now considered the best choice. The arguments are quite complex and are summarized elsewhere.[1,2]

---

*The χ^2 distribution mean and standard deviation are both equal to its degrees of freedom. Larger degrees of freedom (number of cells) approximate a symmetric Normal curve.

The Pearson χ^2 statistic is calculated as:

$$\chi^2 = \sum \frac{(O - E)^2}{E}$$

where O = the observed number in each cell, and E = the expected number in each cell.

The expected number in each cell is that expected if there were no differences between groups so that the ratio of outcome 1 to outcome 2 is the same in each group. Thus for outcome 1, we would expect $(a + b)/N$ as the ratio in each group, the expected number for group A is $([a + b])/N \times [a + c])$, and the expected number for group B is $([a + b])/N) \times [b + d])$. All four expected numbers are calculated and the χ^2 is then the sum of the four $[(O - E)^2]/E$ terms.

The **degrees of freedom** is equal to: (number of rows −1) × (number of columns −1). In a 2×2 table, given fixed row and column totals, there is only free choice for one of the inner numbers because, in doing so, the others are calculated by subtraction. The degrees of freedom was $(2-1)(2-1) = 1$. Thus, in a 2×2 table, the result is compared to known values of the χ^2 distribution at 1 degree of freedom.

For example, consider a clinical trial investigating the effect of pre-operative β–blocker therapy in patients at risk of myocardial ischaemia (Example 6.1).

Example 6.1 An observational study of 20 patients at risk of myocardial ischaemia. Group A is receiving β–blockers, whereas group B is not. The outcome of interest is myocardial ischaemia

Observed:

	Group A	Group B	Row total
Ischaemia	5	12	17
No ischaemia	15	8	23
Column total	20	20	40

Expected (if there was no difference between groups):

	Group A	Group B	Row total
Ischaemia	8.5	8.5	17
No ischaemia	11.5	11.5	23
Column total	20	20	40

χ^2 = (12.25/8.5) + (12.25/8.5) + (12.25/11.5) + (12.25/11.5) = 5.013

The *P* value can be obtained in a χ^2-table in a reference text and is equal to 0.025, and so one would reject the null hypothesis. Thus, patients in group A had a statistically significant lower rate of myocardial ischaemia.

The χ^2 distribution is actually a continuous distribution and yet each cell can only take integers. When the total number of observations is small, the estimates of probabilities in each cell become inaccurate and the risk of **type I error** increases. It is not certain how large N should be, but probably at least 20 with the expected frequency in each cell at least

5. When the expected frequencies are small, the approximation of the χ^2 statistic can be improved by a continuity correction known as **Yates' correction**. The formula is:

$$\chi^2 = \sum \frac{(|O - E| - 0.5)^2}{E}$$

In Example 6.1, the continuity corrected χ^2 is:

$$\chi^2 = (9/8.5) + (9/8.5) + (9/11.5) + (9/11.5) = 3.68$$

This has an associated P value of 0.055 and one would accept the null hypothesis! Yates' correction is considered by some statisticians to be an overly conservative adjustment. It should be remembered that the χ^2 test is an approximation and the derived P value may differ from that obtained by an exact method. We stated above that the Pearson χ^2 test may not be the best approach and this is more so if small numbers of observations are analysed. If there are multiple categories it may be useful to combine them so that the numbers in each cell are greater. With small numbers in a 2×2 table, the best approach is to use Fisher's exact test.

Fisher's exact test

This is the preferred test for 2×2 tables described above. It calculates the probability under the null hypothesis of obtaining the observed distribution of frequencies across cells, or one that is more extreme. It does not assume random sampling and instead of referring a calculated statistic to a sampling distribution, it calculates an **exact probability**. The test examines all the possible 2×2 tables that can be constructed with the same marginal totals (i.e. the numbers in the cells are different but the row and column totals are the same). One can think of this as analogous to the problem of working out all the possible combinations of heads and tails if one tosses a coin a fixed number of times. The probability of obtaining each of these tables is calculated. The probability of all tables with cell frequencies as uneven or more extreme than the one observed is then added to give the final P value. This test was not common before the use of computers because the calculation of probability for each cell was arduous. After constructing all possible tables, the probability of each table is:

$$P = \frac{(a + b)!(c + d)!(a + c)!(b + d)!}{N!a!b!c!d!}$$

Where ! denotes factorial.

In Example 6.1, the P value for Fisher's exact test is 0.054, similar to that obtained using Yates' correction factor, and again we would accept the null hypothesis. Current statistical packages are able to calculate Fisher's exact test and it seems logical to use the exact probability rather than approximate χ^2 tests. Further discussion can be found elsewhere.[1,2]

Analysis of larger contingency tables

If there are more than two groups and/or more than two categories, one can construct larger contingency tables. However, if there are more than two categories, it is often the case that some rank can be assigned to the categories (e.g. excellent, good, poor) and tests such as the **Mann–Whitney U test** may be more appropriate (see Chapter 5).[3] An alternative is to use a variation of χ^2 known as the χ^2 **test for trends**.[4] This test will give a smaller P value if the variation in groups is due to a trend across groups.[4]

The analysis of larger tables can also be carried out using the Pearson χ^2 test as indicated above, with more cells contributing to the test statistic. The result is referred to the χ^2 distribution at $(m-1)(n-1)$ **degrees of freedom**, if there are m rows and n columns. For a *4 × 3* table there are $3 \times 2 = 6$ degrees of freedom. All cells should have an expected frequency greater than 1 and 80% of the cells should have an expected frequencies of at least 5. If this is not the case, it is better to combine some of the categories to have a smaller table.

In the analysis of a large table, for example two categories in three groups, a significant result on χ^2 testing will not indicate which group is different from the others. It is not appropriate to partition the 2×3 table into several 2×2 tables and perform **multiple comparisons**. Three 2×2 tables are possible and a test on each table at the original α may give a spuriously significant result. One approach is to do an initial χ^2 test and, if P is less than 0.05, perform separate tests on each pair using a **Bonferroni correction** for multiple comparisons.[5]

The binomial test

The **binomial distribution** was briefly described in Chapter 2. Data that can only assume one of two groups are called **dichotomous** or **binary data**. Thus, if the proportion in one group is equal to p, then in the other it will be $1 - p$. The binomial test can be used to test whether a sample represents a known dichotomous population.[1] It is a one-sample test based on the binomial distribution. A **normal approximation** based on the z **test** can be used for large samples.[1]

The binomial test could test whether a single study site in a multi-centred trial had a similar mortality to that obtained from the entire study population.

McNemar's chi-square test

McNemar's χ^2 test is used when the frequencies in the 2×2 table represent **paired** (dependent) samples. The null hypothesis is that the paired proportions are equal. The paired contingency table is constructed such that groups A and Y pairs that had an event (outcome 1) would be

Table 6.2 A 2×2 contingency table for paired groups

	Group Y: Outcome 1	Group Y: Outcome 2	Row totals
Group A: Outcome 1	a	b	$a + b$
Group A: Outcome 2	c	d	$c + d$
Column totals	$a + c$	$b + d$	$a + b + c + d = N$

counted in the a cell, those pairs that did not have an event (outcome 2) would be counted in the d cell, and the respective pairs with an event at only one period in cells b and c (Table 6.2).

Groups A and Y denote either **matched pairs** of subjects, or a single group of patients in a **before and after** treatment design. The calculation of McNemar's χ^2 is different from that described above for the Pearson χ^2.[1] The value of the McNemar's χ^2 is referred to the χ^2 distribution with 1 degree of freedom. There is a continuity correction similar to Yates' correction and an exact version of the test that is similar to the Fisher's exact test. If available, the exact test is preferred.

For example, if we had used the group A patients ($n = 20$) described in Example 6.1, but on this occasion had then given them a new treatment, such as low molecular weight heparin, so that we now label them as pre-treatment (group A) and post-treatment (with heparin, group Y), we would get the following table (Example 6.2), still preserving the same distribution of outcomes after each treatment.

Example 6.2 A randomized controlled trial of low molecular weight heparin (LMWH) in 20 patients at risk of myocardial ischaemia who are receiving β-blockers. The outcome of interest is myocardial ischaemia

	Group Y (post-LMWH): Ischaemia	Group Y (post-LMWH): No ischaemia	Row totals
Group A (pre-LMWH): Ischaemia	3	2	5
Group A (pre-LMWH): No ischaemia	9	6	15
Column totals	12	8	20

The McNemar P value is 0.065 (using SPSS V9.0 software). The conclusion from this small before and after study is that LMWH is not effective in the prevention of myocardial ischaemia in patients receiving β-blockers.

The Cochran Q test can be used if there are more than two groups.[1]

Risk ratio and odds ratio

The *P* value derived from a χ^2 statistic does not indicate the *strength* of an association. As clinicians, we are usually interested in how much more likely an outcome will be when a treatment is given or a risk factor is present. This can be described by the **risk ratio** (also known as **relative risk**) and it can be calculated from a 2×2 table (Table 6.3). It is equal to the proportion of patients with a defined outcome after an exposure to a risk factor (or treatment) divided by the proportion of patients with a defined outcome who were not exposed. If exposure is not associated with the outcome, the risk ratio is equal to one; if there is an increased risk, the risk ratio will be greater than one; and if there is a reduced risk, the risk ratio will be less than one.

Because accurate information concerning all patients at risk in a retrospective case-control study is not available (because sample size is set by the researcher), incidence rate and risk cannot be accurately determined, and the **odds ratio** is used as the estimate of the risk ratio (Table 6.3). It is equal to the ratio of the odds of an event in an active group divided by the odds of an event in the control group. It is a reasonable estimate of risk when the outcome event is uncommon (say, < 10%). If the outcome event occurs commonly, the odds ratio tends to overestimate risk.[6] Odds ratios are mostly used in case-control studies that investigate uncommon events.

The risk ratio and odds ratio can be expressed with **95% confidence intervals** (CI).[7] If this interval does not include the value of 1.0, then the association between exposure and outcome is significant (at $P < 0.05$). These methods not only tell you if there is a significant association, but also how strong this association is.

For example, data from Example 6.1 can be reanalysed using these methods (Example 6.3); note that the axes have been switched.

Table 6.3 In prospective cohort studies and clinical trials the risk ratio is equal to the risk of an outcome when exposed compared to the risk when not exposed. For retrospective case-control studies (outcome 'yes' = cases, outcome 'no' = controls), the value for the denominator is unreliable and so the odds ratio is used as an estimate of risk. If an outcome event is uncommon the *a* and *c* cells have very small numbers relative to the *b* and *d* cells, and so the risk ratio can be approximated by the odds ratio, using the fraction *a/b* divided by *c/d*; this can be rewritten as *ad/bc*.

Risk factor (or treatment)	Outcome Yes	No
Yes	*a*	*b*
No	*c*	*d*

Risk ratio $= \dfrac{a/(a+b)}{c/(c+d)}$ Odds ratio $= \dfrac{ad}{bc}$

Example 6.3 An observational study of 20 patients at risk of myocardial ischaemia. Group A is receiving β-blockers, whereas group B is not. The outcome of interest is myocardial ischaemia. The incidence of myocardial ischaemia is high in this study group and so the odds ratio overestimates risk reduction

	Ischaemia	No ischaemia	Row total
Group A β-blocker therapy	5	15	20
Group B No therapy	12	8	20
Column total	17	23	40

$$\text{Risk ratio} = \frac{5/20}{12/20} = \frac{0.25}{0.6} = 0.42$$

$$\text{Odds ratio} = \frac{5 \times 8}{15 \times 12} = \frac{40}{180} = 0.22$$

Thus, using risk ratio, patients receiving β-blocker therapy have a 58% reduction in risk of myocardial ischaemia.

The estimation of risk ratios and odds ratios have been used in epidemiological research for many years where the relationship between exposure to risk factors and adverse outcomes is frequently studied. They are now being used more commonly in anaesthesia research.

For example, Wilson *et al.*[8] investigated the benefits of preoperative optimization and inotropes in patients undergoing major surgery. They randomized 138 patients to receive adrenaline, dopamine or control (routine care). There was a significant reduction in the proportion of patients who had complications in the dopamine group compared with those in the control group. The risk ratio (95% CI) was 0.30 (0.11–0.50), indicating a significant 70% reduction in risk.

Number needed to treat

A risk ratio describes how much more likely it is for an event to occur, but this information is limited unless we consider the baseline level of risk, or **incidence rate**. An increase in risk of a very rare event is still very rare! Thus the change in **absolute risk** is of clinical importance. This is the difference in the probabilities of an event between the two groups. If an event has an incidence of 12% and risk is reduced by 33% (i.e. risk ratio 0.67), then the expected incidence will be 8%; this gives an absolute risk reduction of 4%, or 0.04. If the baseline incidence were 60%, a 25% risk reduction would result in an absolute risk reduction of 15%, or 0.15.

The **number needed to treat (NNT)** is the reciprocal of the absolute risk reduction.[9,10] It describes the number of patients who need to be treated in order to avoid one adverse event. Thus an absolute risk reduction of 0.04 translates to a NNT of 25 (1/0.04) – about 25 patients need to be treated in order to avoid one adverse event. An absolute risk reduction of 0.15 translates to a NNT of 6.7.

For example, data from Example 6.3 can be used to calculate a NNT of 2.9, suggesting that two or three patients need to be treated with β-blockers in order to prevent one patient from having myocardial ischaemia.

For example, Lee *et al.*[11] investigated the use of acupuncture/ acupressure to prevent postoperative nausea and vomiting. They performed a **meta-analysis** of all relevant trials and found that acupuncture/acupressure were better than placebo at preventing early vomiting in adults, with an RR (95% CI) of 0.47 (0.34–0.64). If the incidence of early vomiting is 35% (proportion = 0.35), then these results suggest that acupuncture/acupressure, with an RR of 0.47, would reduce the proportion to 0.17, or an absolute risk reduction of 0.18 (incidence decreased from 35% to 17%). The NNT, or reciprocal of the absolute risk reduction (1/0.18), is 5.5. Therefore, it can be concluded that five to six adult patients need to be treated in order to prevent one patient from vomiting.

A 95% CI can also be estimated for the NNT. It is calculated as the reciprocals of the two 95% confidence limits of the absolute risk reduction.[10]

Mantel–Haenszel test

If a group response is affected by more than one variable, then it may be of interest to determine the relative impact that each of the variables may have on a group outcome. The Mantel–Haenszel χ^2 test can be used to analyse several grouping variables (i.e. it is a **multivariate test**) and so can adjust for **confounding**.[12,13] It stratifies the analysis according to the nominated confounding variables and identifies any that affect the primary outcome variable. If the outcome variable is dichotomous, then **logistic regression** can be used (see Chapters 7 and 8). Both these tests are used most often in outcome studies where there may be several independent (predictor) variables. They can therefore calculate **adjusted odds ratios.**

Kappa statistic

Kappa (κ) measures the agreement between two observers when both are rating the same variable on a categorical scale.[1,14] The κ statistic describes the amount of agreement beyond that which would be due to chance.[14] The difference between the observed proportion of cases in which the raters agree and the proportion expected by chance is divided by the maximum difference possible between the observed and expected proportions, given the marginal totals. The formula for the κ statistic is:

$$\kappa = \frac{A - E}{1 - E}$$

where A = the proportion of times the raters agree, and E = the proportion of agreement expected by chance.

A value of 1.0 indicates perfect agreement. A value of 0 indicates that agreement is no better than chance and the null hypothesis is thus $\kappa = 0$. A κ value of 0.1–0.3 can be described as mild agreement, 0.3–0.5 as moderate agreement, and 0.5–1.0 as excellent agreement. The value of κ can be transformed and tested for statistical significance.[1]

A common situation where kappa is used in anaesthesia studies is to measure agreement between researchers when recording data in clinical trials. Reproducibility is a very important issue in clinical research. For example, Higgins *et al.*[15] developed a risk score from their cardiac surgical database. They measured the reliability of their research nurses data coding and entry by measuring agreement with a sample of reabstracted data checked by study physicians. The kappa statistics were 0.66–0.99, indicating very good agreement, and this supported the validity of their study.

References

1. Siegal S, Castellan NJ Jr. Nonparametric Statistics for the Behavioral Sciences 2nd ed. McGraw-Hill, New York 1988.
2. Ludbrook J, Dudley H. Issues in biomedical statistics: analysing 2 × 2 tables of frequencies. *Aust NZ J Surg* 1994; **64**:780–787.
3. Moses LE, Emerson JD, Hosseini H. Analyzing data from ordered categories. *N Engl J Med* 1984; **311**:442–448.
4. Altman DG. Practical Statistics for Medical Research. Chapman & Hall, London 1991, pp261–264.
5. Bland JM, Altman DG. Multiple significance tests: the Bonferroni method. *Br Med J* 1995; **310**:170.
6. Egger M, Smith GD, Phillips AN. Meta-analysis: principles and procedures. *BMJ* 1997; **315**:1533-1537.
7. Morris JA, Gardner MJ. Calculating confidence intervals for relative risks, odds ratios, and standardised ratios and rates. In: Gardner MJ, Altman DG. Statistics with Confidence – Confidence Intervals and Statistical Guidelines. *British Medical Journal*, London 1989, pp1–63.
8. Wilson J, Woods I, Fawcett J *et al.* Reducing the risk of major elective surgery: randomised controlled trial of preoperative optimisation of oxygen delivery. *BMJ* 1999; **318**:1099–1103.
9. Laupacis A, Sackett DL, Roberts RS. An assessment of clinically useful measures of the consequences of treatment. *N Engl J Med* 1988; **318**:1728–1733.
10. Cook RJ, Sackett DL. The number needed to treat: a clinically useful measure of treatment effect. *BMJ* 1995; **310**:452–454.
11. Lee A, Done ML. The use of nonpharmacologic techniques to prevent postoperative nausea and vomiting: a meta-analysis. *Anesth Analg* 1999; **88**:1362–1369.
12. Kuritz SJ, Landis JR, Koch GG. A general overview of Mantel–Haenszel methods: applications and recent developments. *Ann Rev Public Health* 1988; **9**:123–160.
13. Zeiss EE, Hanley JA. Mantel–Haenszel techniques and logistic regression: always examine one's data first and don't overlook the simpler techniques. *Paediatr Perinat Epidemiol* 1992; **6**:311–315.
14. Morton AP, Dobson AJ. Assessing agreement. *Med J Aust* 1989; **150**:384–387.
15. Higgins TL, Estafanous FG, Loop FD, *et al.* Stratification of morbidity and mortality outcome by preoperative risk factors in coronary artery bypass patients: a clinical severity score. *JAMA* 1992; **267**:2344–2348.

7

Regression and correlation

Association vs. prediction	**Non-linear regression**
Assumptions	**Multivariate regression**
Correlation	**Mathematical coupling**
Spearman rank correlation	**Agreement**
Regression analysis	

Key points
- Correlation and regression are used to describe the relationship between two numerical variables.
- Correlation is a measure of association.
- Spearman rank order (rho) is a non-parametric version of the Pearson correlation coefficient.
- Regression is used for prediction.
- Agreement between two methods of measurement can be described by the Bland–Altman approach or the kappa statistic.

Association vs. prediction

There are many circumstances in anaesthesia research where the strength of a relationship between two variables on a numerical scale is of interest. For example, the relationship between body temperature and oxygen consumption. The commonest methods for describing such a relationship are **correlation** and **regression analysis**, yet these are both frequently misunderstood and misused techniques. One of the reasons for this is that they are used in similar circumstances and are derived from similar mathematical formulae. The main distinction between them is the purpose of the analysis.

Usually one of the variables is of particular interest, whereby we wish to determine how well it is related to the other. This variable of interest is called the **dependent variable**, but is also known as the outcome or response variable. The other variable is called the **independent variable**, but is also known as the predictor or explanatory variable.

The first step in correlation and regression analyses should be to plot a **scatter diagram** (this is essential if misleading conclusions are to be avoided). Here, the dependent (outcome) variable is placed on the y-axis and the independent (predictor) variable is placed on the x-axis, and the plotted data represent individual observations of both variables. For example, if we wanted to describe the relationship between body temperature and total body oxygen consumption (VO_2), we would first plot the respective measurements obtained from each individual: 'a scatterplot' (Figure 7.1).

It appears from this scatterplot that VO_2 increases with increasing body temperature. But how can the relationship between them be described in

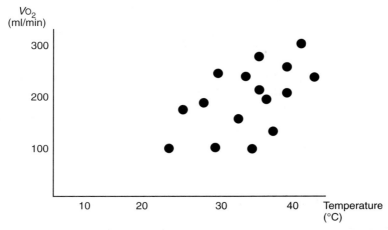

Figure 7.1 A scatterplot of oxygen consumption (VO_2) and temperature. Each data point represents a single observation in each individual patient ($n = 16$)

more detail: how strongly are they associated and, if relevant, are we able to predict VO_2 from body temperature? These are two different questions. The first is described by the **Pearson correlation coefficient** (denoted by r): correlation is a measure of the strength of association. The second question is answered by calculating a regression equation: regression is used for prediction. Thus, one of the major distinctions between correlation and regression is the purpose of the analysis.

Assumptions

Before describing correlation and regression any further, it is important to be aware of their underlying assumptions. First, the relationship between the dependent and independent variable is assumed to be **linear**. This implies that a unit change in one variable is associated with a unit change in the other. The Pearson correlation coefficient describes the degree of scatter of data around a straight line – it is a measure of *linear* association. Two variables can have a strong association but a small correlation coefficient if the relationship is not linear. Similarly, regression is most often used to describe a linear relationship and so simple linear regression is used. This is one of the main benefits of first plotting the data. It allows a visual inspection of the pattern of the scatterplot: if a non-linear relationship is suggested, then alternative techniques can be used which do not assume a linear relationship (some of these are briefly described below).

The data should also be **independent**. This means that each data point on the scatterplot should represent a single observation from each patient. Multiple measurements from each patient should not be analysed using simple correlation or regression analysis as this will lead to misleading conclusions (most often an over-inflated value of *r*, or a misleading regression equation). This is perhaps the most common error relating to correlation and regression in anaesthesia research. **Repeated measures** over time should also not be simply analysed using correlation, as once again this often results in an over-inflated value for *r* (time trends require more advanced statistical methods). Statistical methods are available which can accommodate for such trial designs.[1,2]

These analyses also assume that the observations follow a **normal distribution** (in particular, that for any given value of the independent variable, the corresponding values of the dependent variable are normally distributed). This is known as **homoscedasticity**. If doubt exists, or if the distribution appears non-normal after visualizing a scatterplot, then the data can be transformed (commonly using log-transformation) or a non-parametric method used (e.g. Spearman rank correlation, see below).

Neither correlation nor regression should be used to measure **agreement** between two measurement techniques (see below).

Correlation

The **Pearson correlation coefficient** (*r*) is a measure of how closely the data points on a scatterplot assume a straight line. It is a measure of association. The statistic, *r*, can have any value between −1.0 and + 1.0.* A value of 1.0 describes a perfect positive linear association; a value of −1.0 describes a perfect negative linear association (i.e. as the independent variable increases, the dependent variable decreases). A value of 0 describes no association at all, and this would appear on a scatterplot as a (roughly) circular plot (Figure 7.2). In general, if *r* has an absolute value between 0.2 and 0.4, it may be described as a mild association; a value of 0.4–0.7 would be a moderate association, and 0.7–1.0 a strong association. This distinction is an arbitrary one, however, with the final descriptors of the extent of association being determined more by the intended clinical application.

There is obviously a degree of uncertainty for any calculated value of *r*. This will depend largely on the number of observations (sample size), but is also influenced by various other factors (such as measurement precision, the range of measurements and presence of outliers). The degree of uncertainty can be described by the **standard error** of *r* and its **95% confidence interval**.[3] Perhaps the most useful measure is the value *r²*, the **coefficient of determination**. This is an estimate of how much a change in one variable influences the other (and $1 - r^2$ is the proportion of **variance** yet to be accounted for). For example, from Figure 7.2: 53% $[(0.73)^2]$ of the variability in body weight is explained by age, and 30%

---

*
$$r = \frac{\Sigma(x - \bar{x})\,(y - \bar{y})}{\sqrt{\Sigma(x - \bar{x})^2\,\Sigma(y - \bar{y})^2}}$$

where x = value of independent variable, y = value of dependent variable, and $\bar{x}$ = mean value of x and $\bar{y}$ = mean value of y (several forms of this equation exist).

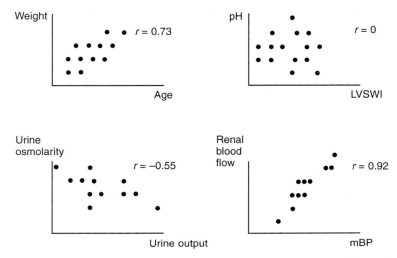

Figure 7.2 Examples of scatterplots demonstrating a variety of correlation coefficients (*r*)

$[(-0.55)^2]$ of the variability in urine osmolarity is explained by a change in urine flow. Knowledge of r^2 therefore has clinical application. It tells us how influential one factor is in relation to another (and perhaps more importantly, the effect of other factors – using $1 - r^2$).

Hypothesis tests can also be applied to correlation; the most common test used is Student's *t*-test.* The *t*-test is used to compare the means of two groups; for correlation, the resultant *P* value describes the likelihood of no correlation ($r = 0$) – it does not describe the strength of that association. Although uncommon, hypothesis tests can also be used to determine if a correlation coefficient is significantly different from some other specified value of *r*.

An important characteristic of correlation is that it is independent of units of measurements. Again, referring to Figure 7.2, the *r* values would not be altered whether body weight was measured in pounds or kilograms, or if mean BP was measured in mmHg or kPa. The value of *r* will, however, be markedly influenced by the presence of outliers (if the range is increased by an outlier there is a tendency for *r* to increase). Similarly, if the range of values is restricted, then *r* will usually be reduced. Data should be randomly selected from a specified target population and measurement precision should be optimized.

A **partial correlation coefficient** can also be calculated. This is an adjusted *r* value which takes into account the impact of a third variable, which may be associated with both the dependent and independent variables (this third variable is called a **covariate**). For example (referring

* $t = r \sqrt{\dfrac{N-2}{1-r^2}}$.

to Figure 7.2), the relationship between age and weight may be influenced by the gender of the patient, or their nutritional status. Similarly, renal blood flow may be affected by changes in cardiac output (which is related to mean blood pressure). If multiple independent (predictor) variables are used to describe a relationship with a dependent (outcome) variable, then a **multiple correlation coefficient** can be calculated (denoted as R) using multivariate regression (see below).

One remaining point should not be forgotten: **association does not imply causation**. A strong association does not, of itself, support a conclusion of cause and effect. This requires additional proof, such as a biologically plausible argument, demonstration of the time sequence (discerning cause from effect) and exclusion of other confounding influences (i.e. a third variable associated with the two variables of interest, that is actually the causative factor).[4] Unfortunately, these issues have been rarely addressed in the anaesthetic literature and this often leads to unsubstantiated conclusions (see also Chapter 11).

Spearman rank correlation

If the distribution of the data is **skewed** (i.e. not normally distributed), then it can be **transformed**, typically using the logarithm of each value to create a more normal distribution to the data so that correlation and regression analyses can then be performed reliably. Alternatively, or if the data are ordinal, a non-parametric version of correlation, such as **Spearman rank correlation** should be used. Because one of the assumptions used in correlation is that the data are normally distributed, then it is also preferable to use Spearman rank correlation when analysing small data sets, say $n < 20$ (as it is difficult to demonstrate a normal distribution with a small number of observations). This calculation is based on the ranking of observations and is denoted by the Greek letter, **rho** (ρ). It is the ordered rank values, rather than the actual values, that are correlated against one another (Table 7.1). In fact, if Spearman's ρ is a similar value to r, then the distribution of the data approximates normal; if not, then it suggests non-normality and the Spearman ρ value should be preferentially used to describe association.

Other aspects of correlation apply equally to both. These include use of the t-test (to derive a P value in order to determine if the correlation is significantly different from zero), standard error, 95% confidence intervals and the coefficient of determination.

There are other non-parametric correlation methods – **Kendall's tau** (τ), **Kendall's coefficient of concordance (W), Cramér coefficient (C), and lambda (L)**. Further details of these methods can be found elsewhere.[5]

Regression analysis

If the aim of the investigation is to predict one variable from another, or at least describe the value of one variable in relation to another, then

Table 7.1 Actual values and their ranking of patient weight and morphine consumption at 24–48 hours after cardiac surgery. These results are a subgroup (n = 23) taken from a study investigating the efficacy of patient-controlled analgesia after cardiac surgery.[6] Spearman's rho (ρ)is calculated by measuring the association between the rank values (if actual values are equal, the rank is calculated as the average between them)

Subject	Weight (kg)	Weight rank	Total dose of morphine (mg)	Morphine rank
1	82	13	13	3
2	86	17	52	19
3	90	9	54	21
4	64	3	29	9
5	83	14	24	7
6	65	4	26	8
7	74	10	38	14
8	53	2	9	1
9	80	12	46	16
10	46	1	19	5.5
11	91	20	53	20
12	69	6	34	12
13	84	15	32	11
14	105	23	30	10
15	78	11	48	17.5
16	73	9	41	15
17	88	18	14	4
18	70	8	36	13
19	97	22	55	22
20	92	21	48	17.5
21	85	16	60	23
22	69	5	12	2
23	89	19	19	5.5

ρ = 0.54 (P = 0.031)

regression analysis can be used. Here the dependent (outcome) variable is again placed on the y-axis of a scatterplot and the independent (predictor) variable is placed on the x-axis. A **line of best fit**, called a **regression line**, can then be calculated using a technique known as the **method of least squares**. This is where the perpendicular difference between each data point and the straight line (this difference is called the residual) is squared and summed – the eventual line chosen is that with the smallest total sum (hence the term 'least squares method' or 'residual sum of squares').

The general formula for the line of best fit is $y = a + bx$, where 'b' is the measure of slope and 'a' is the y-intercept.* For example, referring to our original scatterplot of VO_2 and body temperature (Figure 7.1), a regression line can be derived which enables prediction of VO_2 after measuring body temperature (Figure 7.3). This line is described by the equation, VO_2 (in ml/min) = 6.8 + 6.0 × temp. (in °C). This equation states that for each 1°C increase in temperature there is a 6 ml/min increase in VO_2. From this we are able to predict that if a patient has a body

---

* $b = \dfrac{\Sigma\,(x - \bar{x})\,(y - \bar{y})}{\Sigma\,(x - \bar{x})^2}$ and $a = \bar{y} - b\bar{x}$

temperature of 32°C, then the best estimate for VO_2 would be 199 ml/min, and if their body temperature was 38°C, then $\overset{?}{V}O_2$ would be expected to be 235 ml/min.

Hence regression is a very useful way of describing a linear relationship between two numerical variables. Nevertheless there remains some uncertainty about how accurate this equation is in representing the population: it is unlikely that a derived equation will be able to perfectly predict the dependent variable of interest in the population. This uncertainty can be described by the **standard error** of the slope (b) and its **95% confidence interval**.[3] As the study sample size increases, the standard error of b decreases and so the uncertainty decreases (and the more reliable the regression equation will become). For the population, the general form of the equation is actually $Y' = \beta_0 + \beta_1 X$, where Y' is the predicted value of the dependent variable and β_1 is the slope. Hence, the slope of our sample regression line (b) is an estimate of β_1; β_1 is known as the **regression coefficient**.

In our example (Figure 7.3), the standard error of b can be calculated from a known formula,[3] SE(b) = 2.65. From this we can now calculate a 95% confidence interval for β_1 (after first looking up a t-table, using 14 degrees of freedom [$n - 2$], $t = 2.15$, d.f. = 14): the 95% confidence interval for β_1 is 6.0 ± ([2.15 × 2.65] = 5.7), that is, from 0.3 to 11.7. Because the 95% confidence interval for β_1 does not include the value zero, it is statistically significant at the 5% level ($P < 0.05$). Similarly, a hypothesis test can be performed to test whether a value of β_1 is equal to zero by dividing the value of b by its standard error and looking up a t-table (degrees of freedom = n – 2). Because the level of uncertainty increases the further we are from the mean value of x (our independent variable), the width of the 95% confidence interval increases towards the extreme values. For this reason, 95% confidence intervals for a regression line are curved (Figure 7.4).

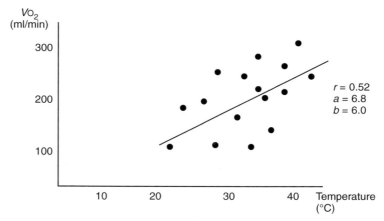

Figure 7.3. A regression line ('line of best fit') for regression of VO_2 on body temperature. Note that the line should not extend beyond the limits of the data (where accurate prediction becomes unreliable)

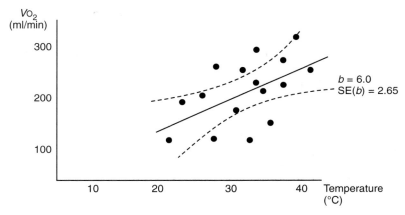

Figure 7.4 A regression line for regression of V_{O_2} on body temperature, showing the 95% confidence intervals (broken lines)

Just as hypothesis testing can be used to determine whether a regression line (slope) is statistically significant (from zero), two regression lines can also be compared to see whether they differ in their Y-intercept or slope (i.e. do they represent two different populations?).

The difference between a predicted value for y and the actual observed value is known as the **residual**. There are methods available which can analyse the distribution of the residuals across a range of values for X in order to determine if the data are normally distributed. The residuals can also be used to describe the '**goodness of fit**' of a regression equation, or '**model**' (i.e. does it predict well?).

The assumptions stated earlier for correlation are also important for regression. However, it is not necessary for the independent (predictor) variable to be normally distributed. It is important to remember that the scale of measurement in regression analysis determines the magnitude of the constants (a and b) in the regression equation, and so units should be clearly stated.

Other, non-linear versions of regression can be used (the above is called simple linear regression). These obviously do not plot a straight line through the scatterplot.

Non-linear regression

An example of non-linear regression is the common classical pharmacokinetic problem of fitting a polyexponential curve to drug concentration–time data.[7] Specialized pharmacokinetic programs are usually used to determine an exponential function that has minimal sum of squares for a set of data points.

Because drug concentrations may vary by several orders of magnitude, and variance is proportional to the concentration, a differential weighting factor is often used for each data point in determining the regression estimates. Several polyexponential solutions are possible and a variety of criteria (e.g. Schwarz, Akaike) can be used to determine the most likely model. Rather than fit individual curves with polyexponential equations, it is becoming common nowadays to carry out population pharmacokinetic modelling that combines all the data points in one overall regression analysis.[8]

The calculation of quantal dose–response curves is another example of the use of non-linear regression. In this case a procedure known as **probit analysis** is often used. In quantal dose–response experiments, several doses of a drug are chosen and the observed response must be dichotomous. (For a log dose–response curve, the doses are best chosen so that the logarithm of the doses are approximately equally spaced.) At each dose, a number of subjects are exposed to the drug and the response observed.

For example, in a comparison of thiopentone requirements between pregnant and non-pregnant patients,[9] the numbers of patients found to be unconscious at each dose was determined (Table 7.2 and Figure 7.5).

The shape of the dose–response curve is expected to be sigmoid and thus the raw proportions of responses in each group must undergo an appropriate transformation. In the **probit transformation**, the proportion responding (y) is transformed using the inverse of the cumulative standard normal distribution function.[10] The basis for this is that a cumulative normal distribution curve is sigmoid in shape. In the **logit transformation,** the proportion responding (y) is transformed using the natural log of the odds ratio: $\ln(y/[1 - y])$. Either transformation can be used and they give similar results. The probit analysis procedure also provides methods to compare the median potency (ED_{50}), and parallelism of two curves, as well as providing confidence limits for the likelihood of response at any dose.

With graded dose-response curve data, a common related method of analysis is to model the data points to fit a sigmoid E_{max} model (i.e. the Hill equation):

$$\frac{E}{E_{max}} = \frac{[D]^{\gamma}}{[D]^{\gamma} + EC_{50}^{\gamma}}$$

where E = effect, E_{max} = the maximum effect, $[D]$ = the drug concentration EC_{50} = the concentration yielding 50% of maximal effect, and γ describes the slope of the curve.

Table 7.2 Number of patients (n = 10) with hypnosis at different doses of thiopentone [10]

Dose (mg/kg)	Non-pregnant	Pregnant
2.0	0	1
2.4	1	5
2.8	4	6
3.3	7	8
3.8	7	10
4.5	10	10
5.3	10	10

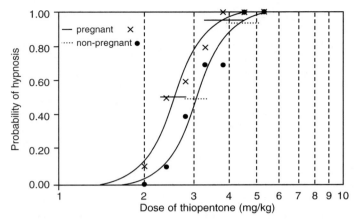

Figure 7.5 Dose–response curves in pregnant and non-pregnant women. The 95% confidence intervals for ED_{50} and ED_{95} are displayed, slightly offset for clarity. Data points are the original proportions in groups of 10 patients

Multivariate regression

Multiple linear regression is a more complex form of regression used when there are several independent variables, using the general form of the equation, $Y' = \beta_0 + \beta_1 X_1 + \beta_2 X_2 + \ldots$

Using this method, many **independent (predictor) variables** can be included in a model, in order to predict the population value of the **dependent (outcome) variable**. It is not necessary for the independent variables to be normally distributed, nor even continuous.

For example, Boyd *et al.*[11] measured arterial blood gases and gastric tonometry (intramucosal pHi) in 20 ICU patients. As part of their analyses, they used multivariate linear regression to describe the relationship between pHi (their dependent variable) and a number of cardiorespiratory (independent) variables. They found mild negative associations with heart rate ($r = -0.29$), systolic pulmonary artery pressure ($r = -0.25$), diastolic pulmonary artery pressure ($r = -0.22$) and blood lactate ($r = -0.36$). Because they also found a strong correlation between blood base deficit and pHi ($r = 0.63$), they concluded that routine blood gas measurements could be used instead of gastric tonometry. Interestingly, they have recently reanalysed their data and included the variable $(Pr\text{-}Pa)CO_2$, the gap between gastric mucosal and arterial carbon dioxide tensions.[12] They found that $(Pr\text{-}Pa)CO_2$ was not correlated with arterial blood gas data and so may be a unique measure of splanchnic perfusion.

Stepwise regression analysis is a type of multivariate analysis used to assess the impact of each of several (independent) variables separately, adding or subtracting one at a time, in order to ascertain whether the addition of each extra variable increases the predictive ability of the equation (model) – the '**goodness of fit**'. It does this by determining whether there has been an increase in the overall value of R^2 (where R = multiple correlation coefficient).

For example, Wong and Chundu used stepwise multiple linear regression to describe factors associated with metabolic alkalosis after paediatric cardiac surgery.[13] Here, the dependent variable was arterial pH, and several patient characteristics and biochemical measures were included as independent variables. They found that patient age and serum chloride concentration were the only significant (negative) associations with arterial pH, and explained 42% of the variability in postoperative arterial pH (i.e. R^2 = 0.42). They concluded that chloride depletion may be a factor in the pathogenesis of metabolic alkalosis in that population.

Analysis of covariance is a combination of regression analysis and analysis of variance (used to compare the mean values of two or more groups), that adjusts for baseline confounding variables (also known as covariates). This method can be used when several groups being compared have an imbalance in potentially important baseline characteristics which may influence the outcome of interest. Here the relationship between each baseline factor and the endpoint of interest is first determined, leading to an adjusted comparison (i.e. so that the groups are 'equalized' before comparison).

Logistic regression is a type of regression analysis used when the outcome of interest is a **dichotomous** (**binary**, or yes/no) **categorical variable**. It generates a probability of an outcome from 0 to 1, using an exponential equation.* This technique is commonly used in outcome studies in anaesthesia and intensive care, where the outcome of interest is a dichotomous variable – typically an adverse event or mortality.[14] As with multivariate linear regression, a number of independent (predictor) variables can be included in the equation, so that their specific effect on outcome can be adjusted according to the presence of other variables. Each independent (predictor) variables may be included in the equation in a stepwise method (one at a time), or all entered together.

If any of the independent variables are also dichotomous, then their relationship to the outcome of interest can be expressed by the **risk ratio**, or its estimate, **odds ratio** (OR) (see Chapter 6). Because this is a multivariate technique, logistic regression can be used to calculate an **adjusted OR**. The OR is the exponential of the regression coefficient (i.e. OR for the factor x_1 is equal to $e^{\beta 1}$).

For example, Kurz *et al.*[15] investigated the potential relationship between postoperative wound infection and various perioperative factors (including maintenance of normothermia) in patients having abdominal surgery. Because wound infection is a dichotomous categorical variable, they used multivariate logistic regression. They found there was a significant association between postoperative wound infection and smoking (OR 10.5), as well as with perioperative hypothermia (OR 4.9).

---

*
$$P = \frac{1}{1 + e^{-w}}$$; it can also be expressed as: OR = e^w

where OR = odds ratio, $w = \beta + \beta_1 x_1 + \beta_2 x_2 + \dots$, and P = probability of outcome.

This means that smokers were approximately 10.5 times more likely to have a postoperative wound infection (compared to non-smokers), and patients who developed hypothermia were 4.9 times more likely (compared to those who were normothermic).

It should be stressed that a number of equations, or 'models', may be developed from a data set using multivariate (linear or logistic) regression analysis. How the final model is constructed depends partly on the choice of independent variables and their characteristics (as numerical, ordinal or categorical data).[16] There may be other (unknown) variables that may have a significant impact on the outcome of interest.[17] Development of a reliable predictive model requires assistance from a statistician experienced in multivariate regression techniques, because of the potential problems with, for example, correlation (**co-linearity**) and **interaction** of variables. But it also requires involvement of an experienced clinician, as the predictor variables ultimately chosen in the model must be reliable and clinically relevant. These predictor variables are often considered as 'risk factors'. Further discussion of these issues can be found in Chapter 8.

Mathematical coupling

If two variables have a mathematical relationship between them, then a spurious relationship can be calculated using correlation. This is known as mathematical coupling and overestimates the value of r.[18] This is also a common error in anaesthesia research, as many endpoints of interest are actually derived (as indices) from another measured variable(s). For example, oxygen delivery (DO_2) is a term derived from a measurement of cardiac output and oxygen content (which in turn is calculated from a measurement of haemoglobin concentration, arterial oxygen saturation and tension).* This is commonly calculated along with VO_2.† Hence, both VO_2 and DO_2 share several values in their derivation. It has been a frequent error to describe the relationship between VO_2 and DO_2 using correlation and regression analysis, with most authors finding an r value of approximately 0.75, and so concluding, possibly falsely, that not only is VO_2 strongly associated with DO_2, but is also dependent on DO_2 (i.e. 'supply-dependence').[19]

Another common situation is where one variable includes the value of the other variable – this is an additive mathematical relationship. An example would be describing the relationship between an initial urine output (say over the first 4 h) and that over 24 h (i.e. 0–4 h and 0–24 h). Clearly the fact that the 24-hour urine volume includes the first 4-hour urine volume will ensure a reasonable degree of association – in this example mathematical coupling can be avoided by excluding the first 4-hour volume from the 24-hour measurement (i.e. 0–4 hours and 4–24 hours). Mathematical coupling should always be considered when one or both variables has been derived from other measurements.

*DO_2 = CO × (Hb × 1.34 × SaO_2 + PaO_2 × 0.003).
†VO_2 = CO × [Hb × 1.34 × (SaO_2 – SvO_2) + (PaO_2 – PvO_2) × 0.003]

Agreement

How well two measurement techniques agree is a common question in anaesthesia and intensive care: comparing two methods of measuring cardiac output, arterial (or mixed venous) oxygen saturation, extent of neuromuscular blockade, depth of anaesthesia, etc. Although correlation is the correct method for measuring the association between two numerical variables, and regression can be used to describe their relationship, they should not (generally) be used to describe agreement between two measurement methods.[20,21] In nearly all situations two methods used to measure the same variable will have very close correlation – but they may not have useful clinical agreement! As an illustration, if two methods differ by a constant amount (which may be quite large) they will have excellent correlation, but poor agreement.

To describe the agreement between two measurement techniques, the average between them (considered the 'best guess') and their difference are first calculated.[20] The average is then plotted against the difference; this plot is sometimes referred to as a **Bland–Altman plot** .[21] The mean difference between measurement techniques is referred to as the **'bias'** and the standard deviation of the difference is referred to as the **'precision'**. The bias is an estimate of how closely the two methods agree on average (for the population), but does not tell us how well the

Table 7.3 Assessing the agreement between two methods of measuring arterial carbon dioxide tension (PCO_2, mmHg) in 20 patients (after Myles *et al.*[22]) The raw data are presented, along with the calculated bias, precision and limits of agreement

Laboratory $LabCO2$	Paratrend-7 $P7CO_2$	Average PCO_2 $(LabCO_2 + P7CO_2)/2$	Difference between methods $LabCO_2 - P7CO_2$
33	37	35	−4
39	39	39	0
39	34	36.5	5
38	36	37	2
42	42	42	0
41	41	41	0
32	31	31.5	1
37	35	36	2
42	41	41.5	1
39	38	38.5	1
29	29	29	0
33	33	33	0
41	40	40.5	1
32	30	31	2
34	33	33.5	1
39	37	38	2
37	36	36.5	1
31	29	30	2
38	36	37	2
43	41	42	2

Mean difference between methods ('bias') = 1.1 mmHg.
Standard deviation (SD) of difference ('precision') = 1.6 mmHg.
1.96 × SD ('limits of agreement') = 3.1 mmHg.

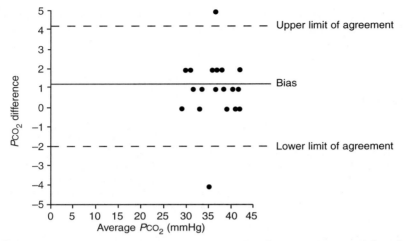

Figure 7.6 Bland–Altman plot of two methods of measuring arterial carbon dioxide tension (P_{CO_2}) (see Table 7.3)

methods agree for an individual. For this we must use the estimate of precision. The precision can be multiplied by 1.96 to calculate the **'limits of agreement'**, which describe where 95% of the data (observed differences) lie. Whether two methods have clinically useful agreement is not determined by hypothesis testing; it is the clinician's impression of the calculated bias and limits of agreement.

For example, two methods for measuring arterial carbon dioxide are the Paratrend 7 intravascular device (Biomedical Sensors, High Wycombe, UK), and a standard laboratory blood gas analyser. These were compared in patients undergoing cardiac surgery[22] and the data recorded after cardiopulmonary bypass are presented in Table 7.3 and Figure 7.6.

If one or both variables are categorical, then the agreement between them can be determined by the **kappa statistic (κ)**. This can be used in situations where, for example, an assessment is made as to whether a disease is present or absent (using either a diagnostic test, predictive score or clinical judgment), and this is compared to another method of assessment. The most common use of the κ statistic is to describe the reliability of two observers' ratings or recordings. The κ statistic describes the amount of agreement beyond that which would be due to chance.[23] A κ value of 0.1–0.3 is sometimes described as mild agreement, 0.3–0.5 as moderate agreement, and 0.5–1.0 as excellent agreement. There are other situations where calculation of positive predictive value, likelihood ratio or risk ratio may be more appropriate (i.e. the chance of a particular outcome, given a test result – see Chapters 6 and 8).

If either of the variables is measured on an ordinal scale (or the question being asked is how well does a measurement technique agree to a previous measurement using the same method?), then the **intraclass**

correlation coefficient can be used.[23] This is a test of reproducibility. The extent of agreement, however, is still best described by the standard deviation of the difference between methods.[20]

References

1. Bland JM, Altman DG. Calculating correlation coefficients with repeated observations: Part I – correlation within subjects. *Br Med J* 1995; **310**:446.
2. Bland JM, Altman DG. Calculating correlation coefficients with repeated observations: Part II – correlation between subjects. *Br Med J* 1995; **310**:633.
3. Altman DG, Gardner MJ. Calculating confidence intervals for regression and correlation. In: Gardner MJ, Altman DG. Statistics with confidence – confidence intervals and statistical guidelines. *British Medical Journal*, London 1989: pp34–49.
4. Sackett DL, Haynes RB, Guyatt GH *et al.* Clinical Epidemiology: A Basic Science for Clinical Medicine, 2nd ed. Little Brown, Boston 1991: pp283–302.
5. Siegel S, Castellan NJ. Nonparametric Statistics for the Behavioural Sciences, 2nd ed. McGraw-Hill International Editions, New York 1988.
6. Myles PS, Buckland MR, Cannon GB *et al.* Comparison of patient-controlled analgesia and conventional analgesia after cardiac surgery. *Anaesth Intens Care* 1994; **22**:672–678.
7. Hull CJ. The identification of compartmental models. In: Pharmacokinetics for Anaesthesia. Butterworth, London 1991: pp187–197.
8. Sheiner LB, Beal SL. NONMEM Users Guide. Division of Clinical Pharmacology, University of California, San Francisco 1979.
9. Gin T, Mainland P, Chan MTV, Short TG. Decreased thiopental requirements in early pregnancy. *Anesthesiology* 1997; **86**:73–78.
10. Finney, D. J. Probit Analysis, 3rd ed. Cambridge University Press, London 1971.
11. Boyd O, Mackay CJ, Lamb G *et al.* Comparison of clinical information gained from routine blood-gas analysis and from gastric tonometry for intramural pH. *Lancet* 1993; **341**:142–146.
12. Rhodes A, Boyd O, Bland JM, Grounds RM, Bennett ED. Routine blood-gas analysis and gastric tonometry: a reappraisal. *Lancet* 1997; **350**:413.
13. Wong HR, Chundu KR. Metabolic alkalosis in children undergoing cardiac surgery. *Crit Care Med* 1993; **21**:884–887.
14. Myles PS, Williams NJ, Powell J. Predicting outcome in anaesthesia: understanding statistical methods. *Anaesth Intensive Care* 1994; **22**:447–453.
15. Kurz A, Sessler DI, Lenhardt R. Perioperative normothermia to reduce the incidence of surgical-wound infection and shorten hospitalization. *N Engl J Med* 1996; **334**:1209–1215.
16. Simon R, Altman DG. Statistical aspects of prognostic factor studies in oncology. *Br J Cancer* 1994; **69**:979–985.
17. Datta M. You cannot exclude the explanation you have not considered. *Lancet* 1993; **342**:345–347.
18. Archie JP. Mathematical coupling of data. A common source of error. *Ann Surg* 1981; **193**:296–303.
19. Myles PS, McRae RJ. Relation between oxygen consumption and oxygen delivery after cardiac surgery: beware mathematical coupling. *Anesth Analg* 1995; **81**:430–431.
20. Bland JM, Altman DG. Statistical methods for assessing agreement between two methods of clinical measurement. *Lancet* 1986; **i**:307–310.

21. Bland JM, Altman DG. Comparing methods of measurement: why plotting difference against standard method is misleading. *Lancet* 1995; **346**:1085–1087.
22. Myles PS, Story DA, Higgs MA *et al.* Continuous measurement of arterial and end-tidal carbon dioxide during cardiac surgery: $P_{a\text{-}ET}CO_2$ gradient. *Anaesth Intensive Care* 1997; **25**: 459–463.
23. Morton AP, Dobson AJ. Assessing agreement. *Med J Aust* 1989; **150**:384–387.

8

Predicting outcome: diagnostic tests or predictive equations

Sensitivity and specificity Prior probability: incidence and prevalence –positive and negative predictive value	Bayes' theorem Receiver operating characteristic (ROC) curve **Predictive equations and risk scores**

Key points
- Sensitivity of a test is the true positive rate.
- Specificity of a test is the true negative rate.
- Positive predictive value is the proportion of patients with an outcome if the test is positive.
- Negative predictive value is the proportion of patients without an outcome if the test is negative.
- A receiver operating characteristic (ROC) curve can be used to illustrate the diagnostic properties of a test on a numerical scale.
- Risk prediction is usually based on a multivariate regression equation.
- A predictive score should be prospectively validated on a separate group of patients.
- Predictive scores are generally unhelpful for predicting uncommon (< 10%) events in individual patients.

Sensitivity and specificity

Diagnostic tests are used to guide clinical practice.[1-3] They are used to enhance a clinician's certainty about what will happen to their patient. The most familiar is a laboratory test or investigation, but many aspects of a clinical examination or patient monitoring should also be considered as diagnostic tests. Predictive equations and risk scores are diagnostic tests. For example, the Mallampati score is commonly used to assess a patient's airway in order to predict difficulty with endotracheal intubation.[4] Clinicians need to know how much confidence should be placed in such tests – are they accurate and reliable?

A diagnostic test usually gives a positive or negative result and this may be correct or incorrect. The accuracy of a diagnostic test can be described by its **sensitivity** and **specificity**. The sensitivity of a test is its true positive rate. The specificity is its true negative rate. Thus the sensitivity and specificity of a test describe what proportion of positive and negative tests results are correct given a known outcome (Figure 8.1).

Common events occur commonly. If a disease is common, and is confirmed by a diagnostic test, then it is very likely to be a true result. Similarly, if a predictive test is positive for an outcome that is common, then it is even more likely to occur. If a test is negative for a common (or expected) event, then the clinician needs to be certain that the chance of

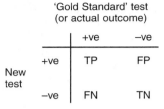

Where   TP = true positive
        FP = false positive
        TN = true negative
        FN = false negative

Sensitivity of the new test = TP/(TP + FN)
Specificity of the new test = TN/(TN + FP)
Positive predictive value of the new test = TP/(TP + FP)
Negative predictive value of the new test = TN/(TN + FN)

Figure 8.1 Sensitivity and specificity, positive and negative predictive value

a false negative result (1–specificity) is extremely low. In most clinical situations a negative test result should be reviewed if clinical suspicion was high. Conversely, a single positive test result for a rare event is unlikely to be true (most positive results will be incorrect).

Prior probability: incidence and prevalence

The value of a diagnostic test in clinical practice does not just depend on its sensitivity and specificity. As stated above, common events can be more confidently predicted and the clinical circumstances in which a test is to be applied must be taken into consideration. Information about prevalence (or incidence) is required. **Prevalence** is the proportion of patients with a disease (or condition of interest) *at* a specified time. **Incidence** is the proportion of patients who develop the disease (or outcome of interest) *during* a specified time. Pre-existing conditions should be described by their prevalence rate, whereas outcomes should be described by their incidence rate. **Prior probability** is a term used interchangeably for prevalence (or incidence, if it is in reference to an expected outcome rate).

Clinical interpretation of diagnostic tests requires consideration of prior probability. This can be done by calculating the **positive predictive value (PPV)** and **negative predictive value (NPV)**. PPV describes the likelihood of disease or outcome of interest *given* a positive test result. NPV describes the likelihood of no disease or avoiding an outcome *given* a negative test result (Figure 8.1). Prior probability is sometimes referred to as the **pre-test risk**; the **post-test risk** refers to either PPV or NPV.

It is common for authors to report optimistic values for PPV and NPV, yet both are dependent on prevalence* – if a disease (or outcome) is

---

*If the test is being used for prediction of outcome (e.g. risk score), then PPV is dependent on its incidence rate.

common, a test (irrespective of its diagnostic utility) will tend to have a high PPV. The same test in another situation where disease prevalence is low will tend to have poor PPV and yet high NPV. Therefore, the context in which the diagnostic test was evaluated should be considered – does the trial population in which the test was developed represent the clinical circumstances in which the test is to be applied? Was there a broad spectrum of patients (of variable risk) studied?[1]

An example of this is electrocardiographic diagnosis of myocardial ischaemia.[2,5] It is generally accepted that ST-segment depression ≥ 1 mm is an indicator of myocardial ischaemia, and with this criterion it has a sensitivity of about 70% and specificity of about 60%.[5] If a 70-year-old man with coronary risk factors is found to have ST-segment depression, then it is very likely that this indicates myocardial ischaemia. But if a 60-year-old woman has the same degree of ST-segment depression, then it remains unlikely that she has myocardial ischaemia.[2,6] This discrepancy can be quantified using PPV and NPV and illustrates the relevance of prior probability (Figure 8.2). In the first case (the elderly man), it could be expected that 60% of such patients (i.e. prior probability 60%) have ischaemic heart disease, but in the second case (the woman), it might only be 10%. If the sensitivity of ECG diagnosis of myocardial ischaemia is 70%, then the PPV for such patients is 74%. The PPV for the woman is only 17%. Rifkin and Hood present a cogent argument describing how the extent of ST-depression should be interpreted according to the perceived risk (prior probability) of myocardial

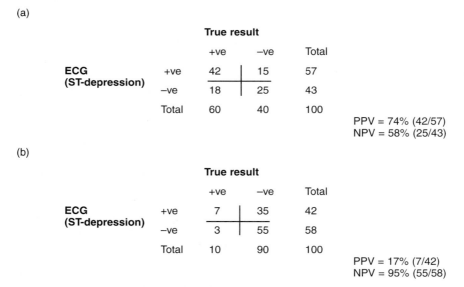

Figure 8.2 The effect of prevalence, or prior probability on PPV and NPV, assuming an ST-segment diagnosis of myocardial ischaemia with sensitivity 70%, specificity 60%: (a) 100 elderly men (prevalence ≈60 %); (b) 100 women (prevalence ≈10%)

ischaemia.[2] PPV can also be calculated by several other methods; one of these is a mathematical formula known as **Bayes' theorem**.

Sensitivity, specificity, PPV and NPV are proportions and so can be described with corresponding **95% confidence intervals**.[7] These are measures of a test's reliability.

Bayes' theorem

Bayes' theorem* is a formula used to calculate the probability of an outcome (or disease), given a positive test result.[2,3] It combines the characteristics of the patient (prior probability), the test (sensitivity) and the test result, to calculate PPV. Bayes' formula states that the PPV is equal to the sensitivity of the test multiplied by the prevalence (or incidence) rate, divided by all those with a positive test (Figure 8.3).

$$P(D^+ \mid T^+) = \frac{P(T^+ \mid D^+) \times P(D^+)}{P(T^+ \mid D^+) \times P(D^+) + P(T^+ \mid D^-) \times P(D^-)}$$

Where P = probability, D^+ = disease (or outcome), D^- = no disease (or outcome), T^+ = test positive, and $P(D^+ \mid T^+)$ = PPV, $P(T^+ \mid D^+)$ = sensitivity.

Figure 8.3 Bayes' theorem

PPV is a **conditional probability**. It is the probability of having the disease (or outcome) *given that* the test was positive. The symbol ' | ' is used to denote that the item to its left presumes the condition to its right.[3] Hence PPV is denoted by $P(D^+ \mid T^+)$. Using this nomenclature, sensitivity can be denoted by $P(T^+ \mid D^+)$ and specificity by $P(T^- \mid D^-)$.

As described above, the utility of a test depends on its accuracy (sensitivity and specificity) and prior probability. If this probability is low, then the ratio of the true positive rate (sensitivity) to the false negative rate (1 –specificity) must be very high in order for the test to be useful in clinical practice. This relationship can be illustrated using a **nomogram**, which illustrates the varying effect of the prior probability and sensitivity of the test, with the likelihood of an outcome.[8] In clinical practice a positive test result usually offers very little extra information for an outcome that is already likely, unless the test is very sensitive and/or specific.

Bayes' theorem can be rearranged to calculate the *odds* of an outcome given a test result – the **likelihood ratio**.[1,2] The prior odds is defined as the odds of an outcome before the test result is known and is the ratio of prior probability to 1 minus prior probability (prevalence/1 –prevalence). Either a positive or negative likelihood ratio can be calculated, according to whether a test result is positive or negative.

A Bayesian approach can also be used to interpret clinical trials.[9] A significant P value for an unexpected event is less likely to be true (i.e.

*Thomas Bayes (1763): 'An essay towards solving a problem in the doctrine of chances'.

lower PPV because of a lower prior probability) than a *P* value that may not be significant (say *P* = 0.11) for an event that had been the main subject of study, or had been demonstrated in previous studies.

The important issue is that *effect size*, not *P* value, is the more important consideration when interpreting clinical trial results. This approach has also been suggested for interim analysis of large trials.[10]

Receiver operating characteristic (ROC) curve

Not all diagnostic test results are simply categorized as 'positive' or 'negative'. Anaesthetists and intensivists are frequently exposed to test results on a numerical scale. Some judgment is required in choosing a cut-off point to denote normal from abnormal (or negative from positive). Laboratory reference ranges are usually calculated from a healthy population, assuming a normal distribution in the population, as mean ± 1.96 standard deviations. Predictive equations, or risk scores, usually have some arbitrary cut-off value, whereby it is considered a higher score denotes higher risk of an adverse outcome ('test positive'). The cut-off value should ideally be selected so that the risk score has greatest accuracy. There is a trade off between **sensitivity** and **specificity** – if the cut-off value is too low it will identify most patients who have an adverse outcome (increase sensitivity) but also incorrectly identify many who do not (decrease specificity).

The change in sensitivity and specificity with different cut-off points can be described by a **receiver operating characteristic (ROC) curve** (Figure 8.4).[3] An ROC curve assists in defining a suitable cut-off point to denote 'positive' and 'negative'. In general, the best point lies at the elbow of the curve (its highest point at the left). However, the final, perhaps most important consideration, is for the intended clinical

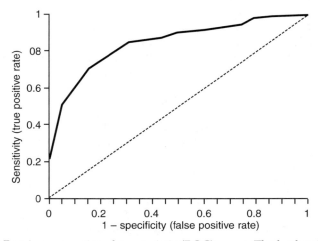

Figure 8.4 Receiver operating characteristic (ROC) curve. The broken line signifies no predictive ability

circumstances to guide the final choice of cut-off point. If the consequences of false positives outweigh those of false negatives, then a lower point on the curve (to the left) can be chosen.

Because an ROC curve plots the relationship between sensitivity and specificity, which are independent of **prevalence**, it will not be affected by changes in prevalence. The slope of the ROC curve represents the ratio of sensitivity (true positive rate) to the false positive rate. The line of equality (slope = 1.0) signifies no predictive ability. The steeper the slope, the greater the gain in PPV.

The area under an ROC curve represents the diagnostic (or predictive) ability of the test. An ROC area of 0.5 occurs with the curve of equality (the line $y = x$) and signifies no predictive ability. Most good predictive scores have an ROC area of at least 0.75. Two or more predictive, or risk, scores can be compared by measuring their ROC areas.[11–13]

For example, Weightman *et al.*[13] compared four predictive scores used in adult cardiac surgery and found they had similar ROC areas (about 0.70) in their surgical population. They concluded that all of the scores performed well when predicting *group* outcome, but would be unreliable for individual patients. This was because adverse outcomes were rare in their study (mortality 3.5%).

Predictive equations and risk scores

Outcome prediction has four main purposes:

- to identify factors associated with outcome (so that changes in management can improve outcome)
- to identify patient groups who are at unacceptable risk (in order to avoid further disability or death, or for resource allocation)
- to match (or adjust) groups for comparison
- to provide the patient and clinician with information about their risk

Identification of low-risk patients (who should not need extensive preoperative evaluation or expensive perioperative care) may save valuable resources for those most at need. Similarly, if patients are at unacceptable risk, whereby expensive resources are not expected to improve outcome, it may be appropriate to deny further treatment. In both of these situations it is imperative that a predictive score is reliable. This is often the case for groups of patients, but less so for the individual. This is a very common problem in anaesthesia because serious morbidity and mortality are rare events and so most 'predictive scores' are not very helpful. **Risk adjustment** is a more accurate way of correcting for baseline differences in clinical studies, or for correcting for 'casemix' when comparing institutions.

Many studies in anaesthesia and intensive care are used to derive a predictive equation or risk score. Information regarding patient demographics, comorbid disease, results of laboratory tests and other clinical data, may be analysed in order to describe their association with eventual patient outcome. This process may identify causative or exacerbating factors, as well as preventive factors.

The simplest method of describing the relationship between a predictor variable and outcome is with one of the familiar **univariate** techniques – for numerical outcomes it may be Student's *t*-test or Mann–Whitney U test; for categorical data it is usually χ^2 or risk ratio calculated from a 2×2 contingency table. Though not essential, these techniques are commonly used during the initial stages of developing a predictive equation or risk score. They act as a screening process in order to identify any possible predictor variables, which are usually chosen as those with $P < 0.05$. These predictor variables are often considered as **'risk factors'**. Univariate techniques cannot adjust for the combined effects of other predictor variables. Hence, with multiple factors, each possibly inter-related, it is necessary to use some form of **multivariate** statistical analysis. These include linear and logistic regression, discriminant analysis and proportional hazards.[14–17]

Regression analysis is used to predict a dependent (outcome) variable from one, or more independent (predictor) variables. **Multiple linear regression** is used when the outcome variable is measured on a numerical scale. **Logistic regression** is used when the outcome of interest is a dichotomous (binary, or yes/no) categorical variable.[15,16] **Discriminant analysis** is used when there are more than two outcome categories (i.e. on a categorical or ordinal scale). **Cox proportional hazards** is used when the outcome is time to an event (usually mortality).[15,18,19] Further descriptions of these methods can be found in Chapters 7 and 9.

Stepwise regression analysis is a type of multivariate analysis used to assess the impact of each of several predictor variables separately, adding or subtracting one at a time, in order to ascertain whether the addition of each extra variable increases the predictive ability of the equation, or *model* – the **'goodness of fit'**. A forward stepwise procedure adds one variable at a time; a backward stepwise procedure removes one variable at a time. It does this by determining whether there has been a significant increase (for a forward procedure) or decrease (for a backward procedure) in the overall value of R^2 (for regression methods, where R = multiple correlation coefficient) or a **goodness of fit** statistic (similar to χ^2).[16,20] R^2 measures the amount of variability explained by the model and is one method of describing its reliability. It is a measure of effect size. $1 - R^2$ is the proportion of variance yet to be accounted for. This process may not necessarily select the most valid, or clinically important, predictor variables.[17] It may also continue to include factors that offer very little additional predictive ability (at the expense of added complexity). An alternative, or complementary, method is to first include known, established risk factors.

A derived equation, or model, is likely to be unreliable if too few outcome events are studied.[15] This may result in spurious factors being identified ('over-fitting' the data) and important ones being missed. The reliability, or precision, of the equation is dependent on the size of the study. The larger the sample the more reliable the estimate of risk. It is recommended that at least ten outcome events should have occurred with each predictor variable in the model.[15,17]

The **regression coefficients**, or weightings, assume a linear gradient between the predictor variable and the outcome of interest. This means that a unit change in the predictor variable will be associated with a unit change in the probability of the outcome. It is best to check for this by visual inspection of the plotted data or stratifying the predictor variables into ordered groups to confirm that the effect is uniform across the range of values. It may be preferable to categorize a numerical predictor variable if this more clearly discriminates different levels of risk.

It must be stressed that a number of equations, or models, may be developed from a data set.[15,17] How the final model is constructed depends partly on the choice of predictor variables and their characteristics, or coding (as numerical, ordinal or categorical data).[15,17] There may be other variables, known or unknown, that may have a significant impact on the outcome of interest.[21] Development of a reliable predictive model requires assistance from a statistician experienced in multivariate techniques, because of the potential problems with, for example, correlation (**co-linearity**) and **interaction** of variables. But it also requires involvement of an experienced clinician, as the predictor variables ultimately chosen in the model must be reliable and clinically relevant.[17]

Because outcome prediction is usually based on a predictive equation developed using multivariate analyses, it will, by virtue of its derivation, be able to predict that original data set well.[14,15,17] Further validation is required before accepting its clinical utility. One method is to split the study population into two, deriving a risk score from the first and testing it on the second. Another method is to prospectively validate it using another data set, or preferably, externally validating the equation, or score, at another institution.[17] **Bootstrapping** is a method of random sampling and replacement from the data set so that multiple samples can be analysed in order to validate the derived model, or risk score.[22] It has been shown to be a more reliable method than split-samples. This method was used recently by Wong *et al.*,[23] when identifying risk factors for delayed extubation and prolonged length of stay with fast-track cardiac surgery.

Wasson *et al.*[14] and others[1,15,17] have described standards for derived predictive scores. They include a clearly defined outcome, clearly defined (objective) risk factors, separation of predictive and diagnostic factors (ideally with blinded assessment of outcome), a clearly defined study population (ideally a wide spectrum of patients) and prospective validation in a variety of settings.[14]

Each of the above multivariate methods derives an equation that predicts the probability of an outcome of interest. Because regression equations are often very complex, it is common to convert them to a risk score for clinical use.[15] The **regression coefficients** (from linear or logistic regression), **odds ratios** (from logistic regression) or **hazard ratios** (proportional hazards) usually form the basis of a numerical score for each risk factor.

Outcome prediction only applies to groups of patients. If a predictive equation or risk score estimates that the risk of postoperative mortality is 42%, this does not mean that a patient with the specified characteristics has a 42% risk of death, only that if 100 similar patients were to proceed with surgery, then 42 would be expected to die postoperatively. We do not know with any certainty, *which* of those patients will survive or die.

One remaining point should not be forgotten: association does not imply causation. For this reason, treatment of identified risk factors may not improve outcome. Just because a strong association is demonstrated, does not, of itself, support a conclusion of cause and effect. This requires added proof, such as a biologically plausible argument, demonstration of the time sequence (discerning cause from effect) and exclusion of other, perhaps unknown, confounding factors.[21,24] For example, amiodarone has been associated with poor outcome after cardiac surgery,[25] yet this may be partly explained by the fact that patients who have been treated with amiodarone are more likely to have poor ventricular function and it may be this confounding factor that explains the poor outcome. This issue could be clarified with a prospective, randomized controlled trial.

Outcome during and after ICU admission has been the subject of many studies. The most familiar are the **APACHE scoring systems**.[26] These were developed because ICU patients frequently suffer multisystem disease and previous risk scores usually focused on a single organ dysfunction or disease. In **APACHE III**, Knaus *et al.*[26] collected data on predictor variables and patient outcome from 26 randomly selected hospitals and 14 volunteer hospitals in the USA. A total of 17 440 patients were studied as a split sample. The first (derivation) group had weights calculated for various chronic disease and physiological variables using logistic regression and these weights were converted into scores. The APACHE III was then prospectively tested on a second (validation) group. A series of regression equations and the APACHE III score are available to calculate the probability of various ICU outcomes.[26] Seneff and Knaus have written an excellent review of several ICU scoring systems.[27]

A good example of a predictive, or risk score is that developed by Higgins *et al.*[28] who collected retrospective data on 5051 patients undergoing coronary artery bypass grafting.[28] They used χ^2 and Fisher's exact test to identify risk factors associated with morbidity and mortality, and also calculated odds ratios to measure the degree of association. Significant risk factors identified by these **univariate** methods were then entered into a **logistic regression** analysis. This enabled **adjusted odds ratios** (for confounding) to be calculated. The final logistic equation, or model, was tested for its predictive ability ('goodness-of-fit') using a test similar to χ^2 (called the **Hosmer–Lemeshow statistic**). It should be noted, that at this stage of their study, they only validated their model on their original data set and so naturally they found their model had good predictive properties. They then used the univariate odds ratios (and 'clinical considerations') to give each significant factor a score of 1 to 6. They also constructed **ROC curves** to compare various versions of their derived clinical severity score. *Importantly*, they then prospectively collected data on a further 4169 patients at their institution and tested their score on this (validation) group. The overall agreement with this new data set was also tested with the Hosmer–Lemeshow statistic. They calculated that if a score of 6 (out of 33) was chosen as a cut-off point for mortality, their score had a sensitivity of 63% and specificity of 86%, and a PPV of 11% and a NPV of 99%. As the authors state, because the PPV was only 11% (i.e. for each 100 patients identified by their score, only 11 actually died postoperatively; the other 89 survived), their score is best to identify low-risk patients as the NPV was 99%.

The bispectral index (BIS) is an EEG-derived estimate of depth of hypnosis.[29] In earlier versions, the manufacturers used multivariate regression to calculate the probability of movement. This was later modified to correlate the BIS with level of hypnosis. In either case, regression analysis was used to construct a range of BIS values that could be used to reflect depth of hypnosis. Thus, BIS is a predictive model. It can be considered to have a certain sensitivity and specificity, and positive and negative predictive value.

References

1. Sackett DL, Richardson WS, Rosenberg W *et al.* Evidence-based Medicine: How to Practice and Teach EBM. Churchill Livingstone, London 1997: pp81–84.
2. Rifkin RD, Hood WB. Bayesian analysis of electrocardiographic exercise stress testing. *N Engl J Med* 1977; **297**:681–686.
3. Metz CE. Basic principles of ROC analysis. *Semin Nucl Med* 1978; **VIII**:283–298.
4. Mallampati SR, Gatt SP, Gugino LD *et al.* A clinical sign to predict difficult intubation: a prospective study. *Can Anaesth Soc J* 1985; **32**:429–434.
5. Carliner NH, Fisher ML, Plotnick GD *et al.* Routine preoperative exercise testing in patients undergoing major noncardiac surgery. *Am J Cardiol* 1985; **56**:51–58.
6. Fleisher LA, Zielski MM, Schulman SP. Perioperative ST-segment depression is rare and may not indicate myocardial ischemia in moderate-risk patients undergoing noncardiac surgery. *J Cardiothorac Vasc Anesth* 1997; **11**:155–159.
7. Gardner MJ, Altman DG. Calculating confidence intervals for proportions and their differences. In: Gardner MJ, Altman DG. Statistics with Confidence. *British Medical Journal*, London 1989: pp28–33.
8. Fagan TJ. Nomogram for Bayes' theorem. *N Engl J Med* 1975; **293**:257.
9. Browner WS, Newman TB. Are all significant p values created equal? The analogy between diagnostic tests and clinical research. *JAMA* 1987; **257**:2459–2463.
10. Brophy JM, Joseph L. Bayesian interim statistical analysis of randomised trials. *Lancet* 1997; **349**:1166–1168.
11. DeLong ER, DeLong DM, Clarke-Pearson DL. Comparing the areas under two or more correlated receiver operating characteristic curves: a nonparametric approach. *Biometrics* 1988; **44**:837–845.
12. Zweig MH, Campbell G. Receiver-operating characteristic (ROC) plots: a fundamental evaluation tool in clinical medicine. *Clin Chem* 1993; **39**:561–577.
13. Weightman WM, Gibbs NM, Sheminant MR *et al.* Risk prediction in coronary artery surgery: a comparison of four risk scores. *MJA* 1997; **166**:408–411.
14. Wasson JH, Sox HC, Neff RK *et al.* Clinical prediction rules: applications and methodological standards. *N Engl J Med* 1985; **313**:793–799.
15. Concato J, Feinstein AR, Holford TR. The risk of determining risk with multivariable models. *Ann Intern Med* 1993; **118**:201–210.
16. Lee J. Covariance adjustment of rates based on the multiple logistic regression model. *J Chronic Dis* 1981; **34**:415–426.

17. Simon R, Altman DG. Statistical aspects of prognostic factor studies in oncology. *Br J Cancer* 1994; **69**:979–985.
18. Cox DR. Regression models and life tables. *J R Stat Soc Series B* 1972; **34**:187–220.
19. Peto R, Pike MC, Armitage P *et al*. Design and analysis of randomized clinical trials requiring prolonged observation of each patient. II. Analysis and examples. *Br J Cancer* 1977; **35**:1–39.
20. Lemeshow S, Hosner DW. A review of goodness-of-fit statistics for use in the development of logistic regression models. *Am J Epidemiol* 1982; **115**:92–98.
21. Datta M. You cannot exclude the explanation you have not considered. *Lancet* 1993; **342**:345–347.
22. Harrell FE, Lee KI, Mark DB. Multivariable prognostic models: issues in developing models, evaluating assumptions and adequacy, and measuring and reducing errors. *Stat Med* 1996; **15**:361–387.
23. Wong DT, Cheng DCH, Kustra R *et al*. Risk factors of delayed extubation, prolonged length of stay in the intensive care unit, and mortality in patients undergoing coronary artery bypass graft with fast-track cardiac anesthesia. A new cardiac risk score. *Anesthesiology* 1999; **91**:936–944.
24. Sackett DL, Haynes RB, Guyatt GH *et al*. Clinical Epidemiology: a Basic Science for Clinical Medicine, 2nd edn. Little Brown, Boston 1991: pp283–302.
25. Mickleborough LL, Maruyama H, Mohammed A *et al*. Are patients receiving amiodarone at increased risk for cardiac operations? *Ann Thorac Surg* 1994; **58**:622–629.
26. Knaus WA, Wagner DP, Draper EA *et al*. The APACHE III prognostic system: risk prediction of hospital mortality for critically ill hospitalized adults. *Chest* 1991; **100**:1619–1639.
27. Seneff M, Knaus WA. Predicting patient outcome from intensive care: a guide to APACHE, MPM, SAPS, PRISM, and other prognostic scoring systems. *J Intens Care Med* 1990; **5**:33–52.
28. Higgins TL, Estafanous FG, Loop FD *et al*. Stratification of morbidity and mortality outcome by preoperative risk factors in coronary artery bypass patients: a clinical severity score. *JAMA* 1992; **267**:2344–2348.
29. Rampil IJ. A primer for EEG signal processing in anesthesia. *Anesthesiology* 1998; **89**:980–1002.

9

Survival analysis

What is survival analysis?
Kaplan–Meier estimate
Comparison of survival curves
  –logrank test
  –Cox proportional hazard model
	The 'hazards' of survival analysis

Key points
- Survival analysis is used when analysing time to an event.
- The Kaplan–Meier method estimates survival using conditional probability, whereby survival depends on the probability of surviving to that point and the probability of surviving through the next time interval.
- Two survival curves can be compared using the logrank test.
- The hazard ratio is the risk of an event compared with a reference group.

What is survival analysis?

Many patients undergoing major surgery, or admitted to intensive care, are at increased risk of early death. Clinical research in these areas often includes measures of outcome such as major morbidity and mortality. But these rates are usually only described at certain points in time (such as in-hospital mortality or 30-day mortality). They ignore other valuable information about exactly *when* the deaths occurred. The actual pattern of death – when, and how many patients die – and its converse, the pattern of survival, are less frequently investigated in anaesthesia and intensive care research. This is particularly so for survival rates over a longer period of time. The statistical analysis of the pattern of survival is known as **survival analysis**.[1,2] The outcome of interest, survival, is treated as a dichotomous (binary, or yes/no) categorical variable and can be presented at any point in time as a proportion.

Although survival analysis is most often concerned with death rates, the outcome of interest may be any **survival event**, such as extubation in ICU, failure of arterial cannulae, or freedom from postoperative nausea and vomiting. The difference, of course, is that in these circumstances complete outcome data on all patients are usually available and so the more familiar comparative statistical tests are most commonly used. However, survival analysis is generally a preferable approach as it provides more clinically relevant information concerning the pattern of the outcome of interest.

If a death rate remains constant, the probability of death over any time period can be estimated (using the Poisson distribution – see Chapter 2). This rarely occurs in clinical practice: usually mortality is high initially, then tapers off. Such rates that vary over time are called **hazard rates**.

Survival, or **actuarial, analysis** is most commonly applied in cancer research, and analysis of outcome after cardiothoracic surgery and organ transplantation. The **mean** time of survival can be a totally misleading statistic, as it will depend on patients' mortality distribution pattern as well as how long they were followed up. The **median** survival time is sometimes used but is only available after more than half the patients have eventually died. Because deaths do not occur in a linear fashion, estimates made over a brief period of time may not reflect the true overall pattern of survival. If some patients have only been in a trial for a few months, we cannot know how many of them will survive over a longer period (say one or two years). Start and finish times (patient recruitment and eventual mortality) are usually scattered. We therefore need a method that accommodates for the incomplete data. The number of patients studied, when they died, and the length of time they have been observed, are crucial data required to describe the pattern of survival.

Because we have information on only those patients who actually died, we do not know how long the remaining patients will survive. These survival times are **'censored'** and the data concerning surviving patients are called censored observations. Censoring removes these individuals from further analysis. Patients who are withdrawn from treatment, or who are lost to follow-up, are also censored observations (at the point they leave the study). Yet the information concerning patients in a trial who have not yet died, or have not yet survived for a specified period, is of some value. After all, we know they have survived for at least that period of time – some of their survival information can be included. Essentially, an estimate is made of the patients' probability of survival, given the observed survival rates in the trial at each time period of interest. Information about the censored data is included (up until they leave or are lost from the trial).

There are two main methods for describing survival data, the **actuarial (life table) method** and the **Kaplan–Meier method**. The actuarial method first divides time into intervals and calculates survival during each of these intervals (censored observations are assumed to have survived to halfway into the interval). The Kaplan–Meier method calculates the probability of survival each time a patient dies. A survival table or graph may be referred to as a **'life table'**. An example, using survival after heart transplantation, is presented in Table 9.1.

Kaplan–Meier estimate

The Kaplan-Meier technique is a non-parametric method of estimating survival and producing a survival curve. The probability of death is calculated when patients die, and withdrawals are ignored (Table 9.2); therefore withdrawals in smaller studies do not have such an effect on calculated survival rates. The Kaplan–Meier method calculates a **conditional probability**: the chance of surviving a time interval can be calculated as the probability of survival up until that time, multiplied by the probability of death during that particular interval. For example, to survive for 15 months, a patient must first survive 12 months, and then three more. The probability of surviving 12 months (using Table 9.2) is

Table 9.1 Survival data after heart transplantation (hypothetical data). The life table describes the observed outcome over two years

Time period	Number of patients alive at the start of each time period	Number of deaths	Alive, but yet to reach next time period (or lost to follow-up)
0–2 mths	74	10	2
2–4 mths	62	4	1
4–6 mths	57	1	1
6–8 mths	55	1	2
8–12 mths	52	1	1
12–16 mths	50	2	3
16–20 mths	45	2	1
20–24 mths	42	0	0
24–30 mths	42	2	1
30–36 mths	39	0	1

0.742, and the probability of survival over the next three months is 0.96; hence the probability of surviving 15 months is $0.742 \times 0.96 = 0.712$.

Changes in probability only occur at the times when a patient dies. The resultant Kaplan–Meier curve is step-like, as a change in the proportion surviving occurs at the instant a death occurs (Figure 9.1). Both **standard error** and **95% confidence intervals** can be calculated.[3] These usually widen over the time period because the number of observations decreases.

Comparison of survival curves

The survival pattern of different patient groups can be compared using their survival curves.[2] This is most commonly applied when comparing two (or more) treatment regimens or different treatment periods (changes over time), or deciding whether various baseline patient characteristics (gender, age groups, risk strata, etc.) can be used to predict (or describe) eventual survival. The most obvious method would be to compare the

Table 9.2 Kaplan-Meier estimates for survival after heart transplantation (using the above hypothetical data)

Month of death	Number of patients (p)	Number of deaths (d)	Probability of death (d/p)	Probability of survival (1–d/p)	Cumulative survival
1	74	10	0.135	0.865	0.865
3	62	4	0.065	0.935	0.809
6	57	1	0.018	0.972	0.786
7	55	1	0.018	0.972	0.764
12	52	1	0.019	0.971	0.742
15	50	2	0.040	0.960	0.712
20	45	2	0.044	0.956	0.681
28	42	2	0.048	0.952	0.648

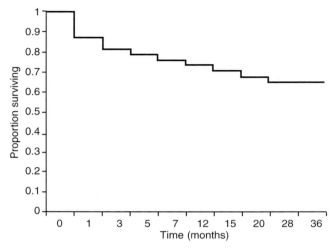

Figure 9.1 Kaplan–Meier survival curve for heart transplantation (see Table 9.2)

survival rates of the groups using standard hypothesis testing for **categorical data** (such as the familiar **chi-square test**). But this is unreliable, as it only depicts the groups at a certain point in time, and such differences between groups will obviously fluctuate. What is needed is a method that can compare the whole pattern of survival of the groups. Various non-parametric tests can be used for this purpose.

One technique is to rank the survival times of each individual and use the **Wilcoxon rank sum test** (survival time is not normally distributed and so the *t*-test would be inappropriate). This method is unreliable if there are censored observations (i.e. patients lost to follow-up or still alive). In these situations, a modification known as the generalized Wilcoxon test can be used (also known as the **Breslow** or **Gehan test**). In general, these tests are uncommonly used because they are not very powerful and so may fail to detect significant differences in survival between groups.

An alternative (and popular) technique is to use the **logrank test**.[2] This is based on the χ^2 test and compares the observed death rate with that expected according to the null hypothesis (the **Mantel–Haenszel test** is also a variation of this). Time intervals are chosen (such as one- or two-month periods) and the number of deaths occurring in each is tabulated. The logrank test then determines the overall death rate (irrespective of group), and compares the observed group death rate with that expected if there was no difference between groups. The results of each time interval are tabulated and a χ^2 statistic is generated. An advantage of the logrank test is that it can also be used to produce an odds ratio as an estimate of risk of death: this is called a **hazard ratio**. A test for trends can also be used, so that risk stratification can be quantified.

For example, Myles *et al.*[4] compared two anaesthetic techniques in patients undergoing cardiac surgery. The time to tracheal extubation was

Table 9.3 Kaplan–Meier estimates for tracheal extubation after coronary artery bypass graft surgery in patients receiving either an enflurane-based (Enf), or propofol-based (Prop) anaesthetic (using data from Myles *et al.*[4])

Time after ICU admission (h)	Number of patients		Number of patients extubated		Probability of extubation		Probability of continued mechanical ventilation		Cumulative proportion still ventilated	
	Enf	*Prop*	*Enf*	*Prop*	*Enf*	*Prop*	*Enf*	*Prop*	*Enf*	*Prop*
0	66	58	0	0	0.00	0.00	1.00	1.00	1.00	1.00
2	66	58	2	4	0.03	0.07	0.97	0.93	0.97	0.93
4	64	54	7	12	0.11	0.22	0.89	0.78	0.86	0.72
6	57	42	9	12	0.16	0.29	0.84	0.71	0.73	0.52
8	48	30	4	3	0.08	0.10	0.92	0.90	0.67	0.47
10	44	27	7	10	0.16	0.37	0.84	0.63	0.56	0.29
12	37	17	11	7	0.30	0.41	0.70	0.59	0.39	0.17
14	26	10	6	3	0.23	0.30	0.77	0.70	0.30	0.12
16	20	7	8	0	0.40	0.00	0.60	1.00	0.18	0.12
18	12	7	5	2	0.42	0.29	0.58	0.71	0.11	0.09
20	7	5	2	0	0.29	0.00	0.71	1.00	0.08	0.09
22	5	5	1	1	0.20	0.20	0.80	0.80	0.06	0.07
24	4	4	0	0	0.00	0.00	1.00	1.00	0.06	0.07

analysed using survival techniques (Table 9.3 and Figure 9.2). This study demonstrated that a propofol-based anaesthetic technique, when compared to an enflurane-based technique, resulted in shorter extubation times. As stated above, survival techniques do not need to be restricted to analysing death rates but can be used to analyse many terminal events of interest in anaesthesia and intensive care research. Because eventual outcome was known for all patients in Myles' study (i.e. there were no

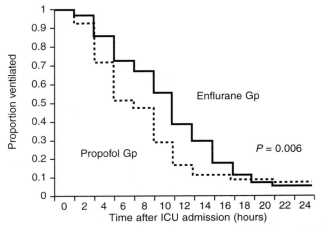

Figure 9.2 Kaplan–Meier survival curves, illustrating tracheal extubation after coronary artery bypass graft surgery in patients receiving either an enflurane-based or propofol-based anaesthetic (see Table 9.3)

censored observations), traditional (non-parametric) hypothesis testing was also employed to compare the median time to extubation.

The **Cox proportional hazards model** is a multivariate technique similar to logistic regression, where the dependent (outcome) variable of interest is not only whether an event occurred, but when.[5] It is used to adjust the risk of death when there are a number of known confounding factors (**covariates**) and therefore produces an adjusted hazard ratio according to the influence on survival of the modifying factors. Common modifying factors include patient age, gender and baseline risk status.

For example, Mangano *et al.*[6] investigated the benefits of perioperative atenolol therapy in patients with, or at risk of, coronary artery disease. They randomized 200 patients to receive atenolol or placebo. Their major endpoint was mortality within the two-year follow-up period. They used the logrank test to compare the two groups and found a significant reduction in mortality in those patients treated with atenolol ($P = 0.019$), principally through a reduction in cardiovascular deaths. They then used the **Cox proportional hazards** method to identify other (univariate) factors that may be associated with mortality. These included diabetes ($P = 0.01$) and postoperative myocardial ischaemia ($P = 0.04$). When these factors were included in a multivariate analysis, only diabetes was a significant predictor of mortality over the two-year period ($P = 0.01$).

The 'hazards' of survival analysis

Comparison of survival data does not need to be restricted to the total period of observation, but can be split into specific time intervals. For example, an early and late period can be artificially constructed for analysis, the definition of these periods being determined by their intended clinical application. This may be a useful exercise if differences only exist during one or other periods, or if the group survival curves actually cross. In general, such arbitrary decisions should be guided by clinical interest, and not be influenced *after* visualization of the survival curves.

Presentation of survival data should include the number of individuals at each time period (particularly at the final periods, where the statistical power to detect a difference is reduced), and survival curves should also include 95% confidence intervals. A comparison of mortality rates at a chosen point in time should not be based upon visualization of survival curves (when the curves are most divergent): this may only reflect random fluctuation and selective conclusion of significance may be totally misleading. Conclusions based upon the terminal (right-hand) portion of a survival curve are often inappropriate, because patients numbers are usually too small. It is common for such curves to have long periods of flatness (i.e. where no patient dies); this should not be interpreted as no risk of death (or 'cure').

In summary, the Kaplan–Meier method is used to estimate a survival curve using conditional probability, the logrank test is used to compare survival between groups, and the Cox proportional hazards method is used to study the effects of several risk factors on survival.

References

1. Peto R, Pike MC, Armitage P *et al.* Design and analysis of randomized clinical trials requiring prolonged observation of each patient. I. Introduction and design. *Br J Cancer* 1976; **34**:585–612.
2. Peto R, Pike MC, Armitage P *et al.* Design and analysis of randomized clinical trials requiring prolonged observation of each patient. II. Analysis and examples. *Br J Cancer* 1977; **35**:1–39.
3. Machin D, Gardner MJ. Calculating confidence intervals for survival time analysis. In: Gardner MJ, Altman DG. Statistics with Confidence – Confidence Intervals and Statistical Guidelines. British Medical Journal, London 1989: pp64–70.
4. Myles PS, Buckland MR, Weeks AM *et al.* Hemodynamic effects, myocardial ischemia, and timing of tracheal extubation with propofol-based anesthesia for cardiac surgery. *Anesth Analg* 1997; **84**:12–19.
5. Cox DR. Regression models and life tables. *J R Stat Soc Series B* 1972; **34**:187–220.
6. Mangano DT, Layug EL, Wallace A *et al.* Effect of atenolol on mortality and cardiovascular morbidity after noncardiac surgery. *N Engl J Med* 1996; **335**:1713–1720.

10

Large trials, meta-analysis, and evidence-based medicine

Efficacy vs. effectiveness Large randomized trials Meta-analysis and systematic reviews	Evidence-based medicine Clinical practice guidelines

Key points
- Stringently designed randomized trials are best to test for efficacy, but lack applicability.
- Large randomized trials are best to test for effectiveness, and so have greater applicability (generalizability).
- Large randomized trials can detect moderate beneficial effects on outcome.
- Meta-analysis combines the results of different trials to derive a pooled estimate of effect.
- Meta-analysis is especially prone to publication bias.
- A systematic review is a planned, unbiased summary of the evidence to guide clinical management.
- Evidence-based medicine optimizes the acquisition of up-to-date knowledge, so that it can be readily applied in clinical practice.
- Clinical practice guidelines are developed by an expert panel using an evidence-based approach.

Efficacy vs. effectiveness

The randomized controlled trial (RCT) is the gold standard method to test the effect of a new treatment in clinical practice. It is a proven method of producing the most reliable information, because it is least exposed to bias.[1–3] Randomization balances known and unknown confounding factors that may also affect the outcome of interest.

Stringently designed RCTs are best to test for **efficacy**, but lack applicability.[4,5] They are conducted in specific patient populations, often in academic institutions, by experienced researchers. They are *explanatory* trials. They commonly exclude patients with common medical conditions or at higher risk. For these reasons their results may not be widely applicable and so they do not necessarily demonstrate **effectiveness** in day-to-day clinical practice. Trials that test effectiveness are also called *pragmatic* trials.[6]

Large RCTs are usually conducted in many centres, by a number of clinicians, on patients who may have different characteristics, and so have greater applicability (generalizability).[2,4,5] Large RCTs are an excellent way of testing for effectiveness.[2,4]

Why we need large randomized trials in anaesthesia*

A good clinical trial asks an important question and answers it reliably.[2,8] In 1984, Yusuf *et al.*[2] explained how large, simple randomized trials can reliably detect moderate effects on important endpoints (e.g. mortality, major morbidity).[2] In part they argued: (a) effective treatments are more likely to be important if they can be used widely, (b) widely applicable treatments are generally simple, (c) major endpoints (death, disability) are more important and assessment of these endpoints can be simple, and (d) new interventions are likely to have only a moderate beneficial effect on outcome. These considerations have fostered the widespread use of large multi-centred RCTs, particularly in the disciplines of cardiology and oncology. Do these issues apply to anaesthesia?

The use of surrogate, or intermediate, outcome measures in anaesthesia is widespread.[9–12] Their inherent weaknesses include uncertain clinical importance, transience, and unconvincing relationships with more definitive endpoints. One of the reasons for studying surrogate endpoints is that more definitive endpoints, such as mortality or major morbidity, are very uncommon after surgery, and anaesthesia is considered to play a small role in their occurrence.[5] Nevertheless, important, moderate effects of anaesthetic interventions are worthy of study, but these require large RCTs in order to be reliable.[3,4,6]

The increasing interest in evidence-based medicine has added a further imperative to conducting reliable clinical trials.[3,5] Small studies can rarely answer important clinical questions. Most improvements in our specialty are incremental, and these require large numbers of patients to be studied in order to have the power to detect a clinically significant difference.[12] McPeek argued 13 years ago that changes in anaesthetic practice should be based on reliable trial evidence that can be generalized to other situations.[4]

Large RCTs are more likely to convincingly demonstrate effectiveness because their treatments are generally widely applicable.[2,4,5] They are usually multi-centred, and perhaps multi-national, in order to maximize recruitment and enable early conclusion. This offers an opportunity to identify other patient, clinician and institutional factors that may influence outcome. These extraneous, potentially confounding factors are more likely to be balanced between groups in large RCTs.[4,13,14] They are therefore less biased and so are more reliable,[4,13,15] with less chance of false conclusion of effect (**type I error**) or no effect (**type II error**).

What is a large trial? This depends on the clinical question. Some will accept trials that study more than 1000 patients, but the more important issue is that the trial should have adequate **power** (> 80%) to detect a true difference for an important primary endpoint.[16,17] Most important adverse outcomes after surgery are rare. For example, the incidence of stroke, renal failure or death after coronary artery surgery is 2–4%, and the incidence of major sepsis after colorectal surgery is 5–10%. In order to

*This has been adapted from an Editorial in *British Journal of Anaesthesia*,[7] published with permission.

Table 10.1 The approximate number of patients needed to be studied (assuming a type I error 0.05 and type II error 0.2)

Baseline incidence	25% improvement with intervention	Number of patients
40%	30%	920
20%	15%	2500
10%	7.5%	5400
6%	4.5%	9300

detect a moderate, but clinically important difference between groups, many thousands of patients are required to be studied (Table 10.1).

There have been some excellent examples of large RCTs in anaesthesia.[18–20] In some of these the investigators selected a high-risk group in order to increase the number of adverse events in the study; this reduced the number of patients required (i.e. with a fixed sample size this equates to a higher incidence rate).

Meta-analysis and systematic reviews

Meta-analysis is a process of combining the results of different trials to derive a pooled estimate of effect and is considered to offer very reliable information.[21–23] Some recent examples in anaesthesia include the effect of ondansetron on postoperative nausea and vomiting (PONV),[24] the role of epidural analgesia in reducing postoperative pulmonary morbidity,[25] and the benefit of acupressure and acupuncture on PONV.[26]

The term **systematic review**, or overview, is sometimes used interchangeably with meta-analysis, but this more aptly describes the complete process of obtaining and evaluating all relevant trials, their statistical analyses, and interpretation of the results. The most well-known is the **Cochrane Collaboration**,[27,28] an Oxford-based group that was established to identify all randomized controlled trials on specific topics. They have several subgroups that focus on particular topics, including acute pain management and obstetrics. An anaesthetic subgroup is being considered (see web-site: www.cochrane-anaesthesia. suite.dk).

Individual trial results can be summarized by a measure of treatment effect and this is most commonly an **odds ratio** (OR) and its **95% confidence interval** (95% CI). The OR is the ratio of odds of an outcome in those treated vs. those not treated. It is a commonly used estimate of risk. An OR of 1.0 suggests no effect; less than 1.0 suggests a reduction in risk, and greater than 1.0 an increased risk. If the 95% CI of the OR exceeds the value of 1.0, then it is not statistically significant at $P < 0.05$ (i.e. it may be a chance finding).

The results (ORs) of individual trials are combined in such a way that large trials have more weight. As stated above, differences in trial characteristics (**heterogeneity**) can obscure this process. For this reason, it is recommended that a **random effects model** be used to combine ORs, whereby the individual trials are considered to have randomly varied results. This leads to slightly wider 95% CI.

Results from each trial can be displayed graphically. The OR (box) and 95% CI (lines) for each subsequent trial are usually displayed along a vertical axis. The size of the box represents the sample size of the trial. The pooled OR and 95% CI for all the trials is represented at the bottom as a diamond, with the width of the diamond representing the 95 CI%. If this pooled result does not cross the value 1.0, it is considered to be statistically significant. A logarithmic scale is often used to display ORs because increased or decreased risk can be displayed with equal magnitude.[23]

For example, Lee and Done[26] investigated the role of acupressure and acupuncture on PONV.[26] They found eight relevant studies and produced a summary diagram (Figure 10.1). The pooled estimate of effect for prevention of early vomiting (expressed as a risk ratio in their study) was 0.47 (95% CI: 0.34–0.64). They did a sensitivity analysis, by separately analysing large and small trials, those of good quality, and those where a sham treatment was included.

The trials included in a meta-analysis should have similar patient groups, using a similar intervention, and measure similar endpoints. Each of these characteristics should be defined in advance. Meta-analysis may include non-randomized trials, but this is not recommended because it obviously weakens their reliability.

Meta-analysis has been criticized,[11,29] and some of its potential weaknesses identified.[16,17,23,30–32] These include **publication bias**

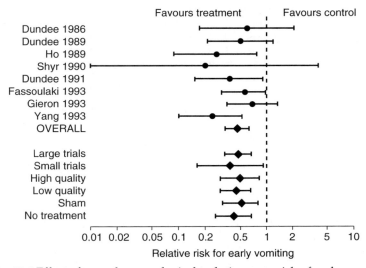

Figure 10.1 Effect of non-pharmacological techniques on risk of early postoperative vomiting in adults • = relative risk for individual study, ♦ = overall summary effect. The control was sham or no treatment. Large trials = n > 50, small trials = $n \le 50$, high-quality studies = quality score > 2, low-quality studies = quality score ≤ 2.

(negative studies are less likely to be submitted, or accepted, for publication), duplicate publication (and therefore double-counting in the meta-analysis), **heterogeneity** (different interventions, different clinical circumstances) and inclusion of historical (outdated) studies.

Despite these weaknesses, meta-analysis is considered a reliable source of evidence.[22,28] There are now established methods to find all relevant trials,[23] and so minimize publication bias. These include electronic database searching, perusal of meeting abstracts and personal contact with known experts in the relevant field. Advanced statistical techniques (e.g. weighting of trial quality, use of a random effects model, funnel plots) and sensitivity analysis can accommodate for heterogeneity[16,21,23,30,31]. The QUOROM statement, a recent review, has formulated guidelines on the conduct and reporting of meta-analyses.[32]

Meta-analyses sometimes give conflicting results when compared with large RCTs.[16,17,29,30] A frequently cited example is the effect of magnesium sulphate on outcome in patients with acute myocardial infarction.[17,21,30,33,34] Many small RCTs had suggested that magnesium improves outcome after acute myocardial infarction and this was the conclusion of a meta-analysis, LIMIT-2, published in 1992.[35] A subsequent large RCT, ISIS-4, disproved the earlier finding.[36]

There have been several explanations for such disagreement.[33,34] But it is generally recognized that positive meta-analyses should be confirmed by large RCTs. Meta-analyses that include one or more large RCTs are considered to be more reliable.[29] Meta-analyses that find a lack of treatment effect can probably be accepted more readily.[11]

The findings of a meta-analysis are sometimes presented as the **number needed to treat** (NNT).[28,37] Here the reciprocal of the absolute risk reduction can be used to describe the number of patients who need to be treated with the new intervention in order to avoid one adverse event. For example, Tramer *et al.*[24] found a pooled estimate in favour of ondansetron , with an OR (95% CI) of approximately 0.75 (0.71–0.83)*. If the incidence of early PONV is 60% (proportion = 0.60), then these results suggest that ondansetron, with an OR of 0.75, would reduce the proportion to 0.45, or an absolute risk reduction of 0.15 (60% to 45%). The NNT, or reciprocal of the absolute risk reduction (1/0.15) is 6.7. Therefore, it can be concluded that six or seven patients need to be treated in order to prevent one patient from having PONV.

Evidence-based medicine

Evidence-based medicine (EBM) has been defined by its proponents as the 'conscientious, explicit and judicious use of current best evidence in making decisions about the care of individual patients'.[28] Although referred to as a new paradigm in clinical care,[15] it could more accurately

---

*The authors calculated odds ratios (as estimates of risk ratios) in terms of a relative benefit, and so we have used the reciprocal to present their results as a relative reduction in PONV (a ratio of benefit of 1.3 became an OR of 0.75).

be described as a simplified approach that optimizes the acquisition of up-to-date knowledge, so that it can be readily applied in clinical practice. As such, EBM formalizes several aspects of traditional practice. The five steps of EBM are:[28]

Step 1. Ask an answerable question
Step 2. Search for evidence
Step 3. Is the evidence valid?
Step 4. Does the evidence apply to my patient?
Step 5. Self-assessment

It teaches how to formulate a specific and relevant question arising from clinical practice, how to efficiently and reliably access up-to-date knowledge ('evidence'), and then reminds us of established critical appraisal skills used to asses the validity of that evidence.

The fourth, and perhaps most important, step is to use clinical expertise in order to determine whether that evidence is applicable to our situation. It is this step that requires clinical experience and judgment, understanding of basic principles (such as pathophysiology, pharmacology and clinical measurement), and discussion with the patient before a final decision is made.[5,15,28] EBM also has a fifth step, asking clinicians to evaluate their own evidence-based practice.

There have been some concerns raised about the application of evidence-based methods in anaesthetic practice.[11,12,38] Some clinicians argue that the principles of EBM are in fact those of good traditional care, and not a new paradigm or approach to clinical practice.[11,38] But the central feature of EBM is its direct application at the bedside (or in the operating suite), with a specific patient or procedure in mind. For this reason, it has direct relevance for us, encourages active learning, and should reduce poor anaesthetic practices not supported by evidence.

What constitutes 'evidence'? Most classifications consider how well a study has minimized bias and rate well-designed and conducted RCTs as the best form of evidence (Table 10.2).[22,39] But it is generally accepted that other trial designs play an important role in anaesthesia research and can still be used for clinical decision-making.[3,5,8,12,28]

Table 10.2 Level of evidence supporting clinical practice (adapted from the US Preventive Services Task Force)

Level	Definition
I	Evidence obtained from a systematic review of all relevant randomized controlled trials
II	Evidence obtained from at least one properly designed randomized controlled trial
III	Evidence obtained from other well-designed experimental or analytical studies
IV	Evidence obtained from descriptive studies, reports of expert committees or from opinions of respected authorities based on clinical experience

More recently, there has been some recognition that the level of evidence (I–IV) is not the only aspect of a study that is of relevance to clinicians when they apply the results in their practice. Thus, the *dimensions* of evidence are all important: level, quality, relevance, strength and magnitude of effect.

Myles *et al.*[22] surveyed their anaesthetic practice and found that 96.7% was evidence based, including 32% supported by RCTs. These results are similar to recent studies in other specialties[39,40] and refute claims that only 10–20% of treatments have any scientific foundation.

The traditional narrative review has been questioned in recent years. Their content is largely dependent on the author(s) and their own experiences and biases. EBM favours the systematic review, as an unbiased summary of the evidence base.[41] These have become more commonly used in anaesthesia research.[24–26,42]

Clinical practice guidelines

Clinical practice guidelines have been developed in order to improve processes or outcomes of care.[5,43,44] They are usually developed by a group of recognized experts after scrutinizing all the available evidence. They generally follow similar strategies to that of EBM, and so the strongest form of evidence remains the randomized controlled trial.

In the past clinical practice guidelines were promulgated by individuals and organizations without adequate attention to their validity.[44] More recently there has been a number of excellent efforts at developing guidelines in many areas of anaesthetic practice.[45,49]

The relationship between the RCT and development of clinical practice guidelines has been explored eloquently by Sniderman.[5] He pointed out that both the RCT and practice guidelines developed by an expert committee can be seen as impersonal and detached. Yet, he suggests, this is also their strength, in that they have transparency and objectivity. Because there is often incomplete evidence on which to develop guidelines, there is a risk of them being affected by the interpretations and opinions of the individuals who make up the expert panel. Sniderman points out that they are also a social process and are exposed to personal opinions and compromise.[5] He suggests that their findings can be strengthened by including a diverse group of experts and not to demand unanimity in their recommendations.

As with EBM, systematic evaluation of published trials can also identify important clinical problems that require further study. Smith *et al.*[49] noted that pain medicine (as with many areas in anaesthesia) is rapidly evolving and so guidelines may become outdated within a few years. The cost and effort to maintain them may be a limiting factor in future developments.

The evaluation of clinical practice guidelines can be biased. Participating clinicians may perform better, or enrolled patients may receive better care or report improved outcomes, because they are being studied. This is known as the **Hawthorne effect**. There are several approaches that can minimize this bias.[44] The gold standard remains the

RCT, but this is often not feasible. Other designs include the crossover trial (where both methods of practice are used in each group at alternate times), or the before-and-after study that includes another control group for comparison.[44]

The management of acute pain has received recent attention.[49] For example, the Australian National Health and Medical Research Council established an expert working party to develop clinical practice guidelines for the management of acute pain. Members of the party scrutinized all relevant studies and rated the level of evidence (levels I–IV) in order to make recommendations.

Anaesthetists gain new knowledge from a variety of sources and study designs.[7,11,12,50] Observational studies can be used to identify potential risk factors or effective treatments. In most cases these findings should be confirmed with an RCT. In some circumstances we are interested in a specific mechanistic question for which a small, tightly controlled RCT testing efficacy may be preferable.[3,12,33,51] Investigation of moderate treatment effects on important endpoints are best done using large RCTs.[2,6]

References

1. Sackett DL, Haynes RB, Guyatt GH, Tugwell P. Deciding on the Best Therapy: A Basic Science for Clinical Medicine. Little Brown, Boston 1991: pp187–248.
2. Yusuf S, Collins R, Peto R. Why do we need some large, simple randomized trials? *Stat Med* 1984; **3**:409–420.
3. Rigg JRA, Jamrozik K, Myles PS. Evidence-based methods to improve anaesthesia and intensive care. *Curr Opinion Anaesthesiol* 1999; **12**:221–227.
4. McPeek B. Inference, generalizability, and a major change in anesthetic practice [editorial]. *Anesthesiology* 1987; **66**:723–724.
5. Sniderman AD. Clinical trials, consensus conferences, and clinical practice. *Lancet* 1999; **354**:327–330.
6. Schwarz D, Lellouch J. Explanatory and pragmatic attitudes in therapeutic trials. *J Chron Dis* 1967; **20**:637–648.
7. Myles PS. Why we need large randomised trials in anaesthesia [editorial]. *Br J Anaesth* 1999; **83**:833–834.
8. Duncan PG, Cohen MM. The literature of anaesthesia: what are we learning? *Can J Anaesthesia* 1988; **3**:494–499.
9. Fisher DM. Surrogate end points: are they meaningful [editorial]? *Anesthesiology* 1994; **81**:795–796.
10. Lee A, Lum ME. Measuring anaesthetic outcomes. *Anaesth Intensive Care* 1996; **24**:685–693.
11. Horan B. Evidence based medicine and anaesthesia: Uneasy bedfellows? *Anaesth Intensive Care* 1997; **25**: 679–685.
12. Goodman NW. Anaesthesia and evidence-based medicine. *Anaesthesia* 1998; **53**:353–368.
13. Rothman KJ. Epidemiologic methods in clinical trials. *Cancer* 1977; **39**:S1771–1775.
14. Ioannidis JPA, Lau J. The impact of high-risk patients on the results of clinical trials. *J Clin Epidemiol* 1997; **50**:1089–1098.
15. Evidence-based medicine working group. Evidence-based medicine: a new approach to teaching the practice of medicine. *JAMA* 1992; **268**:2420–2425.

16. Cappelleri JC, Ioannidis JPA, Schmid CH *et al.* Large trials vs meta-analysis of smaller trials: how do their results compare? *JAMA*1996; **276**:1332–1338.
17. LeLoerier J, Gregoire G, Benhaddad A *et al.* Discrepancies between meta-analyses and subsequent large randomized, controlled trials. *N Engl J Med* 1997; **337**:536–542.
18. Kurz A, Sessler DI, Lenhardt R. The study of wound infection and temperature group. Perioperative normothermia to reduce the incidence of surgical-wound infection and shorten hospitalization. *N Engl J Med* 1996; **334**:1209–1215.
19. Mangano DT, Layug EL, Wallace A *et al.* Effect of atenolol on mortality and cardiovascular morbidity after noncardiac surgery. *N Engl J Med* 1996; **335**:1713–1720.
20. Diemunsch P, Conseiller C, Clyti N *et al.* Ondansetron compared with metoclopramide in the treatment of established postoperative nausea and vomiting. *Br J Anaesth* 1997; **79**:322–326.
21. Pogue J, Yusuf S. Overcoming the limitations of current meta-analysis of randomised controlled trials. *Lancet* 1998; **351**:47–52.
22. Myles PS, Bain DL, Johnson F, McMahon R. Is anaesthesia evidence-based? A survey of anaesthetic practice. *Br J Anaesth* 1999; **82**:591–595.
23. Egger M, Davey–Smith G, Phillips AN. Meta-analysis: principles and procedures. *BMJ* 1997; **315**:1533–1537.
24. Tramer MR, Reynolds DJ, Moore RA, McQuay HJ. Efficacy, dose-response, and safety of ondansetron in prevention of postoperative nausea and vomiting. A quantitative systematic review of randomized placebo-controlled trials. *Anesthesiology* 1997; **87**:1277–1289.
25. Ballantyne JC, Carr DB, deFerrabti S *et al.* The comparative effects of postoperative analgesic therapies on pulmonary outcome: cumulative meta-analyses of randomized, controlled trials. *Anesth Analg* 1998; **86**:598–612.
26. Lee A, Done ML. The use of nonpharmacologic techniques to prevent postoperative nausea and vomiting: a meta-analysis. *Anesth Analg* 1999; **88**:1362–1369.
27. Sackett DL, Oxman AD, eds. Cochrane Collaboration Handbook. The Cochrane Collaboration, Oxford 1997.
28. Sackett DL, Richardson WS, Rosenberg W, Haynes RB. Evidence-based Medicine: How to Practice and Teach EBM. Churchill Livingstone, London 1997.
29. Horwitz RI. 'Large-scale randomized evidence: large, simple trials and overviews of trials': discussion: a clinician's perspective on meta-analyses. *J Clin Epidemiol* 1995; **48**:41–44.
30. Egger M, Smith GD. Misleading meta-analysis. Lessons learned from 'an effective, safe, simple' intervention that wasn't. *BMJ* 1995; **310**:752–754.
31. Moher D, Jones A, Cook DJ *et al.* Does quality of reports of randomised trials affect estimates of intervention efficacy reported in meta-analyses? *Lancet* 1998; **352**:609–613.
32. Moher D, Cook DJ, Eastwood S *et al.* Improving the quality of reports of meta-analyses of randomised controlled trials: the QUORUM statement. *Lancet* 1999; **354**:1896–1900.
33. Woods KL. Mega-trials and management of acute myocardial infarction. *Lancet* 1995; **346**:611–614.
34. Antman EM. Randomized trials of magnesium in acute myocardial infarction: big numbers do not tell the whole story. *Am J Cardiol* 1995; **75**:391–393.
35. Woods KL, Fletcher S, Roffe C, Haider Y. Intravenous magnesium sulphate in suspected acute myocardial infarction: results of the second Leicester

Intravenous Magnesium Intervention Trial (LIMIT-2). *Lancet* 1992; **339**:816–819.

36. ISIS-4 Collaborative Group. ISIS-4: a randomised factorial trial assessing early oral captopril, oral mononitrate, and intravenous magnesium sulphate in 58 050 patients with suspected acute myocardial infarction. *Lancet* 1995; **345**:669–665.
37. Laupacis A, Sackett DL, Roberts RS. An assessment of clinically useful measures of the consequences of treatment. *N Engl J Med* 1988; **318**:1728–1733.
38. Various authors: Evidence-based medicine. *Lancet* 1995, **346**:837–840.
39. Ellis J, Mulligan I, Rowe J, Sackett DL. Inpatient general medicine is evidence based. *Lancet* 1995; **346**:407–410.
40. Howes N, Chagla L, Thorpe M, McCulloch P. Surgical practice is evidence based. *Br J Surg* 1997; **84**:1220–1223.
41. Sheldon TA. Systematic reviews and meta-analyses: the value for surgery. *Br J Surg* 1999; **86**:977–978.
42. Munro J, Booth A, Nicholl J. Routine preoperative testing: a systematic review of the evidence. Health Technology Assessment 1997; 1(12).
43. Lomas J. Words without action? The production, dissemination and impact of consensus recommendations. *Ann Rev Pub Health* 1991; **12**:41–65.
44. Grimshaw JM, Russell IT. Effect of clinical guidelines on medical practice. A systematic review of rigorous evaluations. *Lancet* 1993; **342**:1317–1322.
45. American Society of Anesthesiologists Task Force on Management of the Difficult Airway: practice guidelines for management of the difficult airway. *Anesthesiology* 1993; **78**:597–602.
46. Practice Guidelines for Pulmonary Artery Catheterisation: a report by the American Society of Anesthesiologists Task Force on Pulmonary Artery Catheterisation. *Anesthesiology* 1993; **78**:380–394.
47. ACC/AHA Task Force Report. Special report: guidelines for perioperative cardiovascular evaluation for noncardiac surgery. Report of the American College of Cardiology/American Heart Association Task Force on practice guidelines (Committee on Perioperative Cardiovascular Evaluation for Noncardiac Surgery). *J Cardiothorac Vasc Anesth* 1996; **10**:540–552.
48. Practice guidelines for obstetrical anesthesia: a report by the American Society of Anesthesiologists Task Force on Obstetrical Anesthesia. *Anesthesiology* 1999; **90**:600–611.
49. Smith G, Power I, Cousins MJ. Acute pain – is there scientific evidence on which to base treatment? [editorial] *Br J Anaesth* 1999; **82**:817–819
50. Solomon MJ, McLeod RS. Surgery and the randomised controlled trial: past, present and future. *Med J Aust* 1998; **169**:380–383.
51. Powell-Tuck J, McRae KD, Healy MJR *et al.* A defense of the small clinical trial: evaluation of three gastroenterological studies. *BMJ* 1986; **292**:599–602.

11

Statistical errors in anaesthesia

Prevalence of statistical errors in
  anaesthesia journals
Ethical considerations
How to prevent errors
What are the common mistakes?
  –no control group
  –no randomization
  –lack of blinding
  –misleading analysis of baseline
    characteristics
  –inadequate sample size
  –multiple testing, subgroup analyses and interim analysis
  –misuse of parametric tests
  –misuse of Student's *t*-test
  –repeat ('paired') testing
  –misuse of chi-square – small numbers
  –standard deviation vs. standard error
  –misuse of correlation and simple linear
    regression analysis
  –preoccupation with *P* values
  –overvaluing diagnostic tests and
    predictive equations
A statistical checklist

Key points
• Obtain statistical advice before commencement of the study.
• Consider inclusion of a statistician as a co-researcher.

Prevalence of statistical errors in anaesthesia journals

Advances in clinical practice depend on new knowledge, mostly gained through medical research. We otherwise risk stagnation. Yet conclusions based on poor research, or its misinterpretation, can be even more harmful to patient care. The detailed reporting of medical research usually occurs in any of a large number of peer-reviewed medical journals. Approximately 50% of such published reports contain errors in statistical methodology or presentation.[1–5] These errors are also prevalent in the anaesthetic and intensive care literature.[6–8] Avram et al.[7] evaluated the statistical analyses used in 243 articles from two American anaesthesia journals (*Anesthesiology* and *Anesthesia and Analgesia*) and found common errors included treating ordinal data as interval data, ignoring repeated measures or paired data, uncorrected multiple comparisons, and use of two-sample tests for more than two groups. Goodman[8] surveyed five abstract booklets of the Anaesthesia Research Society (UK) and found that 61 of 94 abstracts (65%) contained errors.

These included failure to identify which statistical tests were used, inadequate presentation of data (to enable interpretation of P value), misuse of standard error and, for negative studies, no consideration of type II error.

Most statistical analyses are performed by researchers who have some basic understanding of medical statistics, but may not be aware of fundamental assumptions underlying some of the tests they employ, nor of pitfalls in their execution. These mistakes often lead to misleading conclusions. On some occasions it is apparent that researchers reproduce a previous study's methodology (including statistical techniques), perpetuating mistakes.

Ethical considerations

As stated in the Preface to this book, Longnecker wrote in 1982, 'If valid data are analyzed improperly, then the results become invalid and the conclusions may well be inappropriate. At best, the net effect is to waste time, effort, and money for the project. At worst, therapeutic decisions may well be based upon invalid conclusions and patients' wellbeing may be jeopardized'.[6] Similar statements have been made by others.[2,9]

Flaws in research design and errors in statistical analysis obviously raise ethical issues. In fact, a poorly designed research project should not be approved by an institutional ethics committee unless it is satisfied that the project is likely to lead to valid conclusions. It would be unethical to proceed. Therefore, **ethical review** should include scientific scrutiny of the research design, paying particular attention to methods of **randomization** and **blinding** (if appropriate), definition of outcome measures, identification of which statistical tests will be applied (and on what data), and a reasonable estimation of how many patients will be required to be studied in order to prove or disprove the hypothesis under investigation. Scrutiny at this early stage will do much to avoid the multitude of errors prevalent in the anaesthetic and intensive care literature.

How to prevent errors

A research paper submitted for publication to a medical journal normally undergoes a peer review process. This detects many mistakes, but remains dependent on the statistical knowledge of the journal reviewers and editor. This can vary. One solution is to include a statistician in the process, but this can delay publication, may be unachievable for many journals and may not avoid all mistakes. Some journals only identify those papers with more advanced statistical methods for selective assessment by a statistician. This paradoxical process may only serve to identify papers that already have statistician involvement (as an author) and miss the majority of papers (which do not include a statistician) that are flawed by basic statistical errors.[2] Statisticians can also disagree on how research data should be analysed and presented, increasing the medical researcher's confusion. Complete, valid presentation of study data can be compromised by a journal's word limit and space constraints. What information to include, and in what form, is perhaps best dictated by the policies of the particular journal (see Table 11.1, at the end of this chapter). This can be found in a journal's 'Advice to Authors' section. If in doubt, direct advice can also be sought from the journal's editor.

The ultimate solution, hopefully addressed in part by this book, is for researchers to further develop their knowledge and understanding of medical statistics. The growing market in introductory texts and attendance of medical researchers at statistical courses would appear to be addressing the problems. Readers should be reassured that most studies can be appropriately analysed using basic statistical tests. The skill, of course, is to know which studies require more advanced statistical methods and assistance from a statistician – this should not be undervalued or resisted. After all, 'specialist' consultation occurs in most other areas of clinical practice! If in doubt, the best habit is to have a low threshold for seeking advice. If this is not available, then advice from an experienced clinical researcher may also be of assistance (although, in our experience, this may only perpetuate mistakes).

It cannot be stressed strongly enough: the best time to obtain advice is *during* the process of study design and protocol development. It is very frustrating to receive a pile of data from an eager novice researcher, which has a multitude of deficiencies. The choice of statistical tests depends on the type of data collected (**categorical, ordinal, numerical**) and the exact hypotheses to be tested (i.e. what scientific questions are being asked). Often the study has not been designed to answer the question. Exactly what data to collect, when, and how, are fundamental components of the research design. This can rarely be corrected after the study is completed!

Where possible, inclusion of a statistician as a co-researcher almost always provides a definitive solution.

What are the common mistakes?

The commonest errors are often quite basic and relate more to research design: lack of a control group, no randomization to treatment groups (or poorly documented randomization) and inadequate blinding of group allocation.[1,2] These can seriously increase the risk of **bias**, making the researcher (and reader) susceptible to misleading results and conclusions. Another common problem is inadequate description of methods (including which statistical tests were used for analysing what data). Some of these issues are addressed in more detail in Chapter 4.

Specifically, we have found that the following errors (or deficiencies) are common in the anaesthetic and intensive care literature:

1. No control group
2. No randomization
3. Lack of blinding
4. Misleading analysis of baseline characteristics (confounding)
5. Inadequate sample size (and type II error)
6. Multiple testing
7. Misuse of parametric tests
8. Misuse of Student's *t*-test
    –paired vs. unpaired
    –one-tailed vs. two-tailed
    –multiple groups (ANOVA)
    –multiple comparisons
9. Repeat ('paired') testing
10. Misuse of chi-square – small numbers
11. Standard deviation vs. standard error
12. Misuse of correlation and simple linear regression analysis
13. Preoccupation with *P* values
14. Overvaluing diagnostic tests and predictive equations.

No control group

To demonstrate the superiority of one treatment (or technique) over another requires more than just an observed improvement in a chosen clinical endpoint. A reference group should be included in order to document the usual clinical course (which may include fluctuating periods of improvement, stability and deterioration). In most situations, a contemporary, equivalent, representative control group should be used. Use of an historical control group may not satisfy these requirements, because of different baseline characteristics, quality or quantity of treatment, or methods used for outcome assessment.

If the control group is given a placebo treatment, then the question being asked is 'does the new treatment have an effect (over and above no treatment)?' This is a common scenario in anaesthesia research which only shows that, for example, an antiemetic is an antiemetic, or an inotrope is an inotrope. Placebo-controlled studies have very little value (other than for detecting adverse events – in which case, the study should be of sufficient size to detect them). If the control group is given an active treatment, then the question being asked is 'does the new treatment have an equal or better effect than the current treatment?' This has more clinical relevance.

It is difficult to detect **'regression to the mean'** unless a control group is included. Regression to the mean occurs when random fluctuation, through biological variation or measurement error, leads to a falsely extreme (high or low) value.[10] This leads to a biased selection, whereby a group has a spuriously extreme mean value, that on re-measurement will tend towards the population mean (which is less extreme). This is a common error if group measurements are not stabilized or if there is no control group.

For example, if a study were set up to investigate the potential benefits of acupressure on postoperative pain control, and patients were selected on the basis that they had severe pain (as measured by VAS on one occasion), then it is likely that VAS measurements at a later time will be lower. Is this evidence of a beneficial effect of acupuncture? It may be a result of the treatment given, but it may also be caused by random fluctuation in pain levels: patients with high levels are more likely to have a lower score on retesting and so the average (group) pain level is much more likely to be reduced.

No randomization

The aim of randomization is to reduce **bias** and **confounding**. All eligible patients should be included in a trial and then randomized to the various treatment groups. This avoids selection bias and increases the **generalizability** of the results. In large trials, randomization tends to equalize baseline characteristics (both known and unknown) which may have an effect on the outcome of interest (i.e. confounding). The commonest method is **simple randomization**, which allocates groups in such a way that each individual has an equal chance of being allocated to any particular group and that process is not affected by previous allocations. This is usually dictated by referring to a table of random numbers or a computer-generated list. Other methods are available which can assist in equalizing groups, such as **stratification** and **blocking** (see Chapter 4). These are very useful modifications to simple randomization, but have been under-used in anaesthesia research.

Knowledge of group allocation should be kept secure (blind) until after the patient is enrolled in a trial, in order to reduce bias. The commonest method is to use sealed, opaque envelopes.

Lack of blinding

It is tempting for the subject or researcher to consciously or unconsciously distort observations, measurement, recordings, data cleaning or analyses. Blinding of the patient (**single-blind**), observer (**double-blind**), and investigator (sometimes referred to as triple-blind) can dramatically reduce these sources of bias. Unblinded studies remain unconvincing. Every attempt should be made to maximize blinding in medical research.

Misleading analysis of baseline characteristics

It is not uncommon for patient baseline characteristics to be compared with hypotheses testing. This is wrong for two major reasons. The first does not alter interpretation of the study, yet remains senseless. If treatment allocation is randomized, then performing significance tests only tests the success of randomization! With a significance level of 0.05, roughly one in 20 comparisons will be significant purely by chance. The second reason is more important and may affect interpretation of results. That is, there may be a *clinically significant difference* between the groups which is not detected by significance testing, yet such an imbalance may have an important effect on the outcome of interest. This is known as **confounding**. Just because 'there was no *statistically significant difference* between the groups' does not imply that there were no subtle differences that may unevenly affect the endpoint of interest. An apparent small (statistically non-significant) difference at baseline for a factor that has a strong effect on outcome can lead to serious confounding.

Authors should certainly describe their group baseline characteristics, consider the possibility of confounding, but not falsely reassure the readers that 'there is no significant difference' between them. This can be interpreted by the reader using clinical judgment, after he/she has been provided with the relevant baseline information.

If an imbalance in baseline characteristics is found to exist at the end of the trial (which may well occur by chance!), there are some advanced **multivariate** statistical techniques available which adjust the results *post hoc* (after the event), taking the **covariate** into account. The simplest method to lessen this problem is to stratify the patients according to one or two important confounding variables (e.g. gender, preoperative risk, type of surgery) before randomizing patients to the respective treatment groups. There are some excellent papers which explore these issues in greater depth.[11–13]

Inadequate sample size

A common reason for failing to find a significant difference between groups is that the trial was not large enough (i.e. did not enrol a sufficient number of patients).[8,14] This is a **type II error**, where the **null hypothesis** is accepted incorrectly. Minimization of this occurrence requires consideration of the incidence rate of the endpoint of interest or, for numerical data, the anticipated mean and variance, along with an estimation of the difference between groups that is being investigated. An approximate sample size can then be calculated (see Chapter 3). Rare outcomes, or small differences between groups, require very large studies. If a study concludes 'no difference' between groups, consideration of the treatment effect size (if any) and likelihood of a type II error should be addressed by the authors.

Multiple testing, subgroup analyses and interim analysis

Multiple comparisons between groups will increase the chance of finding a significant difference which may not be real.[15] This is because each comparison has a probability of roughly one in 20 (if using a **type I error**, or α **value**, of 0.05) of being significant purely by chance, and multiple comparisons magnify this chance accordingly. Multiple testing therefore increases the risk of a type I error, where the null hypothesis is incorrectly rejected. This is often called 'a fishing expedition' or 'data dredging'. A similar problem occurs when multiple subgroups are compared at the end of a trial, or during interim testing while a trial is in progress.[16–18]

The best method to reduce this problem is to perform only a minimal number of preplanned comparisons. If a number of comparisons are to be performed, then the nominal P value for significance can be adjusted according to the number of comparisons made (the **Bonferroni correction**). Several other methods are available when comparing multiple groups with analysis of variance (**Scheffe, Dunnett, Newman-Keuls, Tukey**.) All these methods preserve the overall type I error.

Alternatively, some researchers and statisticians have recognized the conservative nature of such methods (which may increase the risk of a type II error!) and choose to report raw P values, allowing the reader to interpret their significance according to the number of tests performed, whether they were preplanned, and how correlated the endpoints were. Other researchers choose a higher level of significance (commonly $P < 0.01$), recognizing the conservative nature of the Bonferroni correction. One method that accommodates this concern is the **Hochberg** procedure which accepts significance if all P values are < 0.05, but if one is > 0.05, then the next must be < 0.025 to be considered significant.[19] Others suggest that adjustment is unnecessary altogether.[20] Care should be exercised before accepting any conclusions based on multiple comparisons. More often such results should only be used to generate further research targeted at the presumed effects (i.e. they should only be used for hypothesis generation).

If subgroups are identified for further comparisons, then they should at least have clinical application and be defined by their baseline characteristics (not response to treatment). Interpretation of **subgroup analyses** is dependent on the magnitude of the treatment effect, the P value, the consistency of the difference, whether the hypothesis preceded or followed the analysis, whether the subgroup analysis was one of a small number of hypotheses tested and the existence of other published evidence that supports the findings.[16,17]

Readers should be aware of **Simpson's paradox**, where all subgroup analyses reveal significant differences, yet no difference exists overall. This is due to an unequal distribution of confounding baseline characteristics.[21]

There are also several methods available which can adjust for the number of repeated looks at the data during the conduct of a trial (**interim analysis**).[15,18] If a significant difference is observed during one of these comparisons, then the trial may be stopped early. One of these is the **O'Brien–Fleming method**, which unevenly apportions the total type I error according to how many looks at the data are planned. For example, a trial that is to have three interim analyses, can have stopping rules of $P < 0.0001$, $P < 0.004$ and $P < 0.019$, leaving a final P value < 0.043 (for an overall type I error of 0.05).

Misuse of parametric tests

Parametric tests (such as Student's t-test and analysis of variance) have important underlying assumptions, particularly a **normal distribution** of numerical data. This requires specific documentation, and can be achieved by plotting the data and demonstrating a normal distribution, and/or analysing the distribution using a test of goodness of fit (e.g. **Kolmogorov–Smirnov test**). This is unlikely to be satisfactorily achieved with smaller studies (say, $n < 20$). For these, either **data transformation** or non-parametric tests should be used.

In general, parametric tests should only be used to analyse numerical data. Ordinal data is best analysed using non-parametric tests (such as Mann–Whitney U test or Kruskall–Wallis analysis of variance). Some statisticians accept that if the observations have an underlying theoretical continuous distribution, such as pain or perioperative risk, then the data can be considered as continuous, even if measured on an ordinal scale. This argument is most credible for larger studies.[22]

Misuse of Student's t-test

As stated above, it is important to verify assumptions of normality when using the *t*-test, as well as independence of the data and equality of variance (see Chapter 5). The *t*-test can only be used to compare two groups; if more than two groups are being compared, then analysis of variance should be used. If the groups are **independent** (this is the usual situation), then the unpaired *t*-test is used. If the groups are related to one another (i.e. **dependent**), as with comparing a group before and after treatment, then the **paired *t*-test** must be used. In most cases a difference between groups may occur in either direction and so a two-tailed *t*-test is used. If there is a clear, predetermined rationale for only exploring an increase, or a decrease, then a **one-tailed *t*-test** may be appropriate. Unfortunately, a one-tailed *t*-test is usually selected to lower a *P* value so that it becomes significant (which a two-tailed test failed to achieve). This is gravely misleading. A paper using a one-tailed *t*-test should be scrutinized: was there a valid reason for only investigating a difference in one direction, and was this preplanned (before analysing the data)?

Repeat ('paired') testing

If an endpoint is measured on a number of occasions (e.g. measurement of postoperative pain, or cardiac index during ICU stay), then any subsequent measurement, at least in part, is determined by the previous measurement. The amount of individual patient variation over time is much less than that between patients (i.e. **intra-group variance** is lower than **inter-group variance**) and so differences can be more easily detected.

If a group endpoint is measured on two occasions then a **paired *t*-test** (or non-parametric equivalent) can be used. If three or more measurements are made, or two or more groups are to be compared on a number of occasions, then the most appropriate method is to use **repeated measures analysis of variance**. If a significant difference is demonstrated overall, then individual comparisons can be made to identify at which time the differences were significant (adjusting *P* values for multiple comparisons).

An alternative approach is to use summary data that describe the variable of interest over time. This may be the overall mean of repeated measurements, or the area under a curve (with time on the x-axis).[23]

Misuse of chi-square – small numbers

Mathematically, the χ^2 distribution is a continuous distribution and the calculated χ^2 statistic is an approximation of this. When small numbers are analysed, there is an artificial incremental separation between potential values. For this reason, an adjustment factor is needed. For a 2×2 contingency table, where there are only two groups being compared, looking at one dichotomous endpoint, **Yates' correction** should be used. This subtracts 0.5 from each component in the χ^2 equation.* If two or more cells in a 2×2 contingency table *of expected values* have a value less than 5, then **Fisher's exact test** should be used (for larger contingency tables the categories can be collapsed, reducing the number of categories and increasing the number in each). These considerations become less important with large studies.

Chi-square should not be used if the groups are matched or if repeat observations are made (i.e. paired categorical data). **McNemar's test** can be used in these situations.

Standard deviation vs. standard error

In a normal distribution, 95% of data points will lie within 1.96 standard deviations of the mean. **Standard deviation (SD)** is therefore a measure of variability and should be quoted when describing the distribution of sample data.[2,7–9,24] **Standard error** is a derived value† used to calculate **95% confidence intervals**, and so is a measure of precision (of how well sample data can be used to predict a population parameter). Standard error is a much smaller value than SD and is often presented (wrongly) for this reason. It should not be confused with standard deviation, nor used to describe variability of sample data. On some occasions it may be acceptable to use standard error bars on graphs (for ease of presentation), but on these occasions they should be clearly labelled.

It has been suggested that the correct method for presentation of normally distributed sample data variability is mean (SD) and not mean ($\pm$ SD).[25]

Misuse of correlation and simple linear regression analysis

These techniques are used to measure a linear relationship between two numerical variables. The **correlation coefficient** is a measure of *linear* association and **linear regression** is used to describe that linear

$$^*\chi^2 = \sum \frac{(O - E - 0.5)^2}{E}$$

$$^\dagger SE = \frac{SD}{\sqrt{n}}$$

relationship. These analyses assume that the observations follow a normal distribution (in particular, that for any given value of the **independent** [predictor] variable, the corresponding values of the **dependent** [outcome] variable are normally distributed). If doubt exists, or if the distribution appears non-normal after visualizing a scatterplot, then the data can be transformed (commonly using **log-transformation**) or a non-parametric method used (e.g. **Spearman rank correlation**).

The data should also be **independent**. This means that each data point on the scatterplot should represent a single observation from each patient. Multiple measurements from each patient should not be analysed using correlation or regression analysis as this will lead to misleading conclusions. **Repeated measures** over time should also not be simply analysed using correlation.[26]

Variables with a mathematical relationship between them will be spuriously highly correlated because of **mathematical coupling**.[27] Further details can be found in Chapter 7.

Normally a scatterplot should be included to illustrate the relationship between both numerical variables. A regression line should not exceed the limits of the sample data (extrapolation).

Neither correlation nor regression should be used to measure **agreement** between two measurement techniques. Bland and Altman have described a suitable method.[28] As with correlation, multiple measurements from each patient should not be plotted together and treated as independent observations (this is a very common mistake in anaesthesia and intensive care research). Further details can be found in Chapter 7.

Preoccupation with P values

Too much importance is often placed on the actual *P* value, rather than the size of the treatment effect.[8,29] A *P* **value** describes the probability of an observed difference being due to chance alone. It does not describe how large the difference is, nor whether it is *clinically* significant. Importantly, a *P* value is affected by the size of the trial: a highly significant *P* value in a large trial may be associated with a trivial difference, and a non-significant *P* value in a small trial may conceal an effect of profound clinical significance. A *P* value is only a mathematical statement of probability, it ignores the more important information from a trial: how large is the **treatment effect**?

The **95% confidence interval** (CI) for effect describes a range in which the size of the true treatment effect will lie. In general, a large trial will have a small standard error and so narrow 95% CI: a more precise estimate of effect. From this the clinician can interpret whether the observed difference is of clinical importance.

Overvaluing diagnostic tests and predictive equations

Diagnostic tests can be described by their **sensitivity** (true positive rate) and **specificity** (true negative rate). This only tells us what proportion of positive and negative tests results are correct (given a known outcome).

Of greater clinical application is the positive and negative predictive values of the test (**PPV** and **NPV** respectively), which inform us of the likelihood of disease (or adverse outcome) given a test result.[30] It is common for authors to report optimistic values for these indices, yet both are dependent on the prevalence of disease – if a disease (or outcome) is common, any test (irrespective of its diagnostic utility) will tend to have a high PPV. A similar test in another situation where disease prevalence is low will tend to have poor PPV, yet high NPV. Therefore, the context in which the diagnostic test was evaluated should be considered – does the trial population in which the test was developed represent the clinical

---

Table 11.1. A statistical checklist used by the British Medical Journal (after Gardner *et al.*[4])

Design features			
1. Was the objective of the trial sufficiently described?	Yes	Unclear	No
2. Was there a satisfactory statement given of diagnostic criteria for entry to trial?	Yes	Unclear	No
3. Was there a satisfactory statement given of source of subjects?	Yes	Unclear	No
4. Were concurrent controls used (as opposed to historical controls)?	Yes	Unclear	No
5. Were the treatments well defined?	Yes	Unclear	No
6. Was random allocation to treatment used?	Yes	Unclear	No
7. Was the method of randomization described?	Yes	Unclear	No
8. Was there an acceptable delay from allocation to commencement of treatment?	Yes	Unclear	No
9. Was the potential degree of blindness used?	Yes	Unclear	No
10. Was there a satisfactory statement of criteria for outcome measures?	Yes	Unclear	No
11. Were the outcome measures appropriate?	Yes	Unclear	No
12. Was there a power based assessment of adequacy of sample size?	Yes	Unclear	No
13. Was the duration of post-treatment follow-up stated?	Yes	Unclear	No
Commencement of trial			
14. Were the treatment and control groups comparable in relevant measures?	Yes	Unclear	No
15. Was a high proportion of subjects followed up?	Yes	Unclear	No
16. Did a high proportion of subjects complete treatment?	Yes	Unclear	No
17. Were the drop-outs described by treatment/control groups?	Yes	Unclear	No
18. Were side-effects of treatment reported?	Yes	Unclear	No
Analysis and presentation			
19. Was there a statement adequately describing or referencing all statistical procedures used?	Yes		No
20. Were the statistical analyses used appropriate?	Yes	Unclear	No
21. Were prognostic factors adequately considered?	Yes	Unclear	No
22. Was the presentation of statistical material satisfactory?	Yes		No
23. Were confidence intervals given for the main results?	Yes		No
24. Was the conclusion drawn from the statistical analysis justified?	Yes	Unclear	No
Recommendation			
25. Is the paper of acceptable statistical standard for publication?	Yes		No
26. If 'No' to Question 25, could it become acceptable with suitable revision?	Yes		No

circumstances for which the test is to be applied? Was there a broad spectrum of patients studied?

Outcome prediction is sometimes based on a **risk score** or **predictive equation** developed from a large data set using multivariate analyses which, by virtue of its derivation, should be able to predict that original data set well. Such derived tests need to be *externally* validated using other data sets, preferably at other institutions before accepting their clinical utility.

Statistical checklist

The British Medical Journal used a statistical checklist,[4] which is reproduced in Table 11.1.

References

1. Gore SM, Jones IG, Rytter EC. Misuse of statistical methods: critical assessment of articles in BMJ from January to March 1976. *Br Med J* 1977; **1**:85–87.
2. Glantz SA. Biostatistics: how to detect, correct and prevent errors in the medical literature. *Circulation* 1980; **61**:1–7.
3. Altman DG, Gore SM, Gardner MJ, Pocock SJ. Statistical guidelines for contributors to medical journals. *Br Med J* 1983; **286**:1489–1493.
4. Gardner MJ, Machin D, Campbell MJ. Use of check lists in assessing the statistical content of medical studies. *Br Med J* 1986; **292**:810–812.
5. Godfrey K. Statistics in practice. Comparing the means of several groups. *N Engl J Med* 1985; **313**:1450–1456.
6. Longnecker DE. Support versus illumination: trends in medical statistics [editorial]. *Anesthesiology* 1982; **57**:73–74.
7. Avram MJ, Shanks CA, Dykes MHM *et al.* Statistical methods in anesthesia articles: an evaluation of two American journals during two six-month periods. *Anesth Analg* 1985; **64**:607–611.
8. Goodman NW, Hughes AO. Statistical awareness of research workers in British anaesthesia. *Br J Anaesth* 1992; **68**:321–324.
9. Altman DG. Statistics and ethics in medical research, v – analysing data. *Br Med J* 1980; **281**:1473–1475.
10. Yudkin PL, Stratton IM. How to deal with regression to the mean in intervention studies. *Lancet* 1996; **347**:241–243.
11. Altman DG. Comparability of randomised groups. *Statistician* 1985; **34**:125–136.
12. Altman DG, Dore CJ. Randomisation and baseline comparisons in clinical trials. *Lancet* 1990; **335**:149–153.
13. Lavori PW, Louis TA, Bailar JC, Polansky M. Designs for experiments – parallel comparisons of treatment. *N Engl J Med* 1983; **309**:1291–1299.
14. Frieman JA, Chalmers TC, Smith H *et al.* The importance of beta, the type II error and sample size in the design and interpretation of the randomized controlled trial. *N Engl J Med* 1978; **299**:690–694.
15. McPherson K. Statistics: the problem of examining accumulating data more than once. *N Engl J Med* 1974; **290**:501–502.
16. Bulpitt CJ. Subgroup analysis. *Lancet* 1988; **ii**:31–34.

17. Oxman AD, Guyatt GH. A consumer's guide to subgroup analysis. *Ann Intern Med* 1992; **116**:78–84.
18. Geller NL, Pocock SJ. Interim analyses in randomized clinical trials: ramifications and guidelines for practitioners. *Biometrics* 1987; **43**:213–223.
19. Hochberg Y. A sharper Bonferroni method for multiple tests of significance. *Biometrika* 1988; **75**:800–802.
20. Michels KB, Rosner BA. Data trawling: to fish or not to fish. *Lancet* 1996; **348**:1152–1153.
21. Abramson NS, Kelsey SF, Safar P, Sutton–Tyrrell K. Simpson's paradox and clinical trials: what you find is not necessarily what you prove. *Ann Emerg Med* 1992; **21**:1480–1482.
22. Moses LE, Emerson JD, Hosseini H. Statistics in practice. Analyzing data from ordered categories. *N Engl J Med* 1984; **311**:442–448.
23. Mathews JNS, Altman DG, Campbell MJ, Royston P. Analysis of serial measurements in medical research. *Br Med J* 1990; **300**:230–235.
24. Horan BF. Standard deviation, or standard error of the mean? [editorial] *Anaesth Intensive Care* 1982; **10**:297.
25. Altman DG, Gardner MJ. Presentation of variability. *Lancet* 1986; **ii**:639.
26. Bland JM, Altman DG. Calculating correlation coefficients with repeated observations: part II – correlation between subjects. *Br Med J* 1995; **310**:633.
27. Archie JP. Mathematical coupling of data: a common source of error. *Ann Surg* 1981; **193**:296–303.
28. Bland MJ, Altman DG. Statistical methods for assessing agreement between two methods of clinical measurement. *Lancet* 1986; **ii**:307–310.
29. Gardner MJ, Altman DG. Confidence intervals rather than *P* values: estimation rather than hypothesis testing. *Br Med J* 1986; **292**:746–750.
30. Myles PS, Williams NJ, Powell J. Predicting outcome in anaesthesia: understanding statistical methods. *Anaesth Intensive Care* 1994; **22**:447–453.

12

How to design a clinical trial

Why should anaesthetists do research?	Role of the ethics committee
Setting up a clinical trial	(institutional review board)
Data and safety monitoring committee	Informed consent
Phase I–IV drug studies	Successful research funding
Drug regulations	Submission for publication

Key points
- Define the study question(s): what is the aim and study hypothesis?
- Perform a literature review.
- Use a pilot study to test your methods, measurement techniques, and generate preliminary data for consideration.
- Develop a study protocol
    - background
    - aim, hypothesis, endpoints
    - study design
    - define groups, intervention(s)
    - measurements, data recording
    - sample size, statistics (and get advice from a statistician)
    - adverse events, safety monitoring.
- Regulation
    - drug licensing
    - ethics committee approval and informed consent.

In most circumstances medical research consists of studying a **sample** of subjects (cells, animals, healthy humans, or patients) so that inferences can be made about a **population** of interest. Unbiased sample selection and measurement will improve the reliability of the estimates of the population parameters and this is more likely to influence anaesthetic practice.

Laboratory research usually investigates underlying mechanisms of disease or aspects of drug disposition. Clinical research occurs in patients. Epidemiology is the study of disease in populations. Each are important and have their strengths. Most anaesthetists undertaking laboratory research are supervised in an experienced (hopefully well-resourced) environment. Clinical research is undertaken by a broad array of researchers, of variable quality and support, with variable infrastructure, equipment and staffing. This chapter is primarily addressing aspects of clinical research.

The best studies are those that answer important questions reliably.[1,2] The most reliable study design is the **randomized controlled trial**,[2–4] but other designs have an important role in clinical research.[1,5,6] One of the main aims of medical research is to produce convincing study results and conclusions that can ultimately improve patient outcome.

Why should anaesthetists do research?

Identification of a clinical problem, and subsequent development and participation in a study hypothesis, design, conduct, analysis and writing of a research project can be a rewarding experience. Unfortunately much research is poor and co-investigators may have little involvement in its development and conduct.[7,8] Involvement in the processes required to complete a successful research project can teach critical appraisal skills, but these can also be explicitly taught at the undergraduate and postgraduate levels.

Many specialist training schemes demand completion of a research project before specialist recognition is obtained, and consultant appointment or promotion usually includes consideration of research output. Thus there are imperatives to 'do research', despite some having a lack of interest, support or specific training. Cynicism is often generated by those who have had poor research experiences. This should be avoidable. Anaesthetic trainees, and those with an interest in research, should be guided and supported in a healthy, funded and staffed research environment.

Setting up a clinical trial

The major steps involved in setting up a clinical trial are:

1. **Define the study question(s).** Explicitly, what are the aims and significance of the project? Identify a primary endpoint (there may be several secondary endpoints); it should be clearly defined, including under what conditions it is measured and recorded. An essential, often neglected step, is to state the study hypothesis. Ultimately, the study design must be able to answer the hypothesis.
2. **Perform a literature review**. Previous studies may help in designing a new study. What is the current evidence in the literature? What questions remain unanswered? What deficiencies exist in previous studies? In other words, explain why you are doing this study.
3. **Develop a study protocol**.
   (a) background – previous published research, outline why this study should be undertaken
   (b) clear description of aim and hypothesis
   (c) overview of study design (retrospective vs. prospective, control group, randomization, blinding, parallel or crossover design) – a good study design minimizes bias and maximizes precision
   (d) study population, criteria for inclusion and exclusion (define population)
   (e) treatment groups, timing of intervention
   (f) clear, concise data collection, defined times, measurement instruments
   (g) sample size calculation based on the primary endpoint[9,10]
   (h) details of statistical methods – get advice from a statistician
   (i) reporting of adverse events, safety monitoring.

4. **Perform a pilot study**. This is an important and neglected process. The study protocol assumptions and methodologies need to be tested in your specific environment. It is an opportunity to test measurement techniques and generate preliminary data that may be used to reconsider the sample size calculation and likely results. Is the recruitment rate feasible?
5. **Modify and finalize the study protocol**. This should be agreed to and understood by all study investigators.
6. **Satisfy regulations**. Drug licensing and ethics committee approval.

Data and safety monitoring committee

Clinical trials may be stopped early if (a) the superiority of one treatment is so marked that it becomes unethical to deny subsequent patients the opportunity to be treated with it, or (b) one treatment is associated with serious risks.

An independent **data and safety monitoring committee** (DSMC) should be established to monitor large trials, and can advise early stopping of a trial in the above circumstances. They are usually guided by predetermined stopping rules derived from **interim analyses**.[11–13]

Phase I–IV drug studies

New drug compound development can take up to 15 years and cost US$700 million to get to market. Laboratory and animal testing of new drug compounds eventually lead to human testing, which is divided into four phases:

1. **Phase I:** this is the first administration in humans (usually healthy volunteers). The aim is to confirm (or establish) basic drug pharmacokinetic data and obtain early human toxicology data. Phase I trials often only include 20–100 human subjects before moving on to phase II trials.
2. **Phase II:** selected clinical investigations in patients for whom the drug is intended, aimed at establishing a dose–response ('dose-finding') relationship, as well as some evidence of efficacy and further safety.
3. **Phase III:** is full-scale clinical evaluation of benefits, potential risks and cost analyses.
4. **Phase IV:** is post-marketing surveillance involving many thousands of patients.

Pharmaceutical companies usually design and sponsor phase I–III studies. Phase IV studies are mostly designed and conducted by independent investigators.

Drug regulations

Most countries have restrictions on the administration and research of new drugs in humans (Table 12.1). There are established **good clinical**

Table 12.1 Websites for government agencies responsible for new drug research or the conduct of clinical trials

Agency	Website
Australia	
Therapeutic Goods Administration (TGA)	www.tga.health.gov.au
Australian Health Ethics Committee (AHEC)	www.health.gov.au/nhmrc/ethics/contents.htm
Canada	
Therapeutic Products Programme (TPP)	www.hc-sc.gc.ca/hpb-dgps/therapeut/
Medical Research Council of Canada	www.mrc.gc.ca
Europe	
European Medicines Evaluation Agency (EMEA)	www2.eudra.org/emea.html
International Conference on Harmonisation (ICH)	www.ifpma.org/ich1.html
United Kingdom	
Department of Health Research and Development	www.doh.gov.uk/research/index.htm
Medicines Control Agency	www.open.gov.uk/mca/mcahome.htm
Committee on Safety of Medicines (CSM)	www.open.gov.uk/mca/csmhome.htm
Medical Research Council (MRC)	www.mrc.ac.uk
United States	
Food and Drug Administration (FDA)	www.fda.gov
Center for Drug Evaluation and Research	www.fda.gov/cder/
National Institutes of Health (NIH)	www.nih.gov
NIH Ethics Program	ethics.od.nih.gov

research practice (GCRP) guidelines for clinical investigators and pharmaceutical companies. These include that a principal investigator should have the relevant clinical and research expertise, there be a formal study protocol, adequate staffing and facilities, ethics approval and informed consent, maintenance of patient confidentiality, maintenance of accurate and secure data, and there be processes to report adverse events.

In Australia, the **Therapeutic Goods Administration** (TGA) of the Commonwealth Department of Health and Aged Care approves new drug trials under one of two schemes:

1. **CTX**: the clinical trials exemption scheme
2. **CTN**: the clinical trials notification scheme.

The CTX scheme requires an expert committee to evaluate all aspects of the drug pharmacology, including potential toxicology (mutagenicity, teratogenicity, organ dysfunction and other reported side-effects) and benefits. The CTN scheme bypasses this evaluation, usually because extensive evaluation has occurred in one of a number of key index countries (Netherlands, New Zealand, Sweden, UK, USA). In this circumstance, the local ethics committee accepts responsibility for the trial.

In the UK, the Licensing Division of the Medicines Control Agency of the Department of Health is responsible for the approval and monitoring of all clinical drug trials. The Secretariat of the Medicines Division of the Department of Health will issue a CTX certificate after evaluation. More extensive phase II–III trials are conducted only after a Clinical Trial Certificate (CTC) is issued and the drug data reviewed by the **Committee on Safety of Medicines** (CSM). The UK, along with most other European countries, is also guided by the **European Medicines Evaluation Agency** (EMEA).

In the USA, the Center of Drug Evaluation and Research, a **Food and Drug Administration** (FDA) body of the Department of Health and Human Services, evaluates new drugs through an **Investigational New Drug** (IND) application. Clinical research can start after 30 days. In Canada, this is overseen by the **Therapeutic Products Programme** (TPP).

In each of these countries there are similar processes required for new therapeutic devices, such as implantable spinal catheters and computer-controlled infusion pumps. Other countries have similar processes which can be found on the world wide web, or via links from websites included in Table 12.1.

The different regulations and standards that have existed in different countries have been an obstacle to drug development and research in humans. This has prompted co-operation and consistency between countries. One of the more significant advances has been the **International Conference on Harmonisation** (ICH) of Technical Requirements for Registration of Pharmaceuticals for Human Use. This includes the regulatory authorities of Europe, Japan and the USA, and the pharmaceutical industry.

Role of the ethics committee (institutional review board)

Advances in medical care depend on medical research, for which laboratory investigation, followed by experimentation on animals and healthy volunteers leads to research on patients. Clinical research should be thoroughly evaluated and supported within an institution so that it has the best chance of being successfully completed and providing reliable results. Poor research leads to misleading results, wastes resources and puts patients at risk, and so is unethical. Ethics committee approval has a role in ensuring good-quality research.[14]

Ethical considerations include the Hippocratic principle of protecting the health and welfare of the individual patient as well as the utilitarian view of the potential benefit for the majority vs. risk to a few. These considerations were explored by earlier investigations into ethical research in humans, such as the **Nuremberg Code** of 1949[15,16] and the **Declaration of Helsinki** in 1964.*[17] Most countries have developed ethical guidelines based on these principles.

* www.cirp.org/library/ethics/helsinki.

In Australia, this is governed by the **National Health and Medical Research Council** (NHMRC) statement on human experimentation and local ethics committees are guided by the NHMRC Australian Health Ethics Committee (see Table 12.1). Medical colleges and associations also have their own ethical guidelines. A similar situation occurs in the UK where the Department of Health has issued guidelines for research within the NHS (including multi-centre research).[18] In the USA, the **National Institutes of Health** (NIH) Ethics Program guides research practices, and in Canada this is guided by the **Medical Research Council of Canada**.

All research involving human beings, either observational or experimental, should include approval through an established ethical review and approval process. This is included in all GCRP guidelines.

Informed consent

Patients should be informed of the nature of the research and be asked to provide informed consent. This requires adequate disclosure of information, potential risks and benefits (if any), competency and understanding, and self-determination.[18–20] Patient confidentiality must be maintained. It should be made clear to patients that they are under no obligation to participate, that they can withdraw from the study at any time, and that refusal or withdrawal will not jeopardize their future medical care.

A key role in the requirement for informed consent for medical research was played by Beecher in the early 1960s.[21] He presented details of 18 studies at a symposium (and later published 22 examples in the *New England Journal of Medicine*) where no patient consent was obtained.[21] Similar examples can still be found in the literature today.[22]

The concept of randomization to different treatment groups is a challenging concept for patients (and some doctors).[23] The ethical principle underlying this process includes the concept of equipoise, whereby the clinician and patient have no particular preference or reason to favour one treatment over another.[18,24] The conflicting roles of researcher and clinician are sometimes difficult to resolve in this situation.[18,23,24] Note that the Declaration of Helsinki includes the words 'The health of my patient will be my first consideration'.

Some have argued that it is not always necessary to obtain consent,[25,26] or that patients are unable to provide truly informed consent,[19,20] or that the clinician is in a better position to consider the relative merits of the research. This paternalistic attitude has been rightly challenged. Madder, in an essay on clinical decision-making, argued cogently that patients are entitled to clear and reasonable information, and that they should be included in decisions regarding their care.[27]

Informed consent can be difficult in anaesthesia research. Patients approached before elective surgery are often anxious and may also be limited by concurrent disease.[23] Feelings of anxiety, vulnerability, confusion or mistrust may dominate their thought processes and restrict their ability to provide informed consent.[20] Alternative randomization methods have been advocated which may address these and other concerns,[28–30] but there is little evidence of benefit.[23]

Obtaining informed consent for clinical trials on the day of surgery has been studied previously[31–33] and is an important consideration given the increasing trend to day-of-admission surgery. Patients generally prefer to be approached for consent well in advance, but still accept recruitment on the day of surgery if approached appropriately (i.e. private setting, adequate time to consider trial information).[31–33] Interestingly, 51% of patients preferred not to know about a trial prior to admission as it only increased their level of anxiety.[32]

Informed consent cannot be obtained in some circumstances. Patients arriving unconscious or critically ill to the emergency department, or those in the intensive care unit who are critically ill, confused or sedated cannot provide informed consent. Government or institutional ethics committees usually provide guidelines in these circumstances.[34]

There are many issues at stake when considering the ethics of research and consent in incompetent subjects. Many argue that such research is important and should be supported. In general consent can be waived if the research has no more than minimal risk to the subjects and it can be demonstrated that the research could not be carried out otherwise.[34] Some institutions consider that a family member or next of kin can provide consent in these circumstances, but this may not be legally binding in many countries. In any case it would be reasonable to inform the patient's family or next of kin of the nature of research so that they have an opportunity to have any concerns or questions answered and be asked to sign an *acknowledgement* form. Under these circumstances the institutional ethics committee accepts greater responsibility until the patient's consent can be sought at a later date (**deferred consent**).

Successful research funding

Peer review funding through major government medical research agencies (e.g. NHMRC, MRC, NIH) is limited to only the top ranked 20% of projects. Other sources of research funds are also available, including from institutions, colleges, associations and benevolent bodies.[35]

Successful funding is more likely if the proposed study addresses an important question that has demonstrable clinical significance (now or in the future). There should be a clearly stated hypothesis and the study design must be capable of answering it. The application must demonstrate that there is minimal bias, and maximal precision and relevance. It should include a sample size calculation and have detailed statistical analyses. The study should be feasible, with demonstrable ability to successfully recruit patients. This is best achieved with pilot or previous study data. A successful track record of the chief investigator (or mentor) is reassuring.

Funding agencies commonly rate applications on a number of criteria. For example, in Australia the NHMRC and the Australian and New

Zealand College of Anaesthetists use the following:

1. Scientific merit
2. Track record
3. Originality
4. Feasibility
5. Design and methods
6. International competitiveness.

The ten most common reasons for failure at NIH are:[36]

1. Lack of original ideas
2. Diffuse, unfocused, or superficial research plan
3. Lack of knowledge of published relevant work
4. Lack of experience in essential methodology
5. Uncertainty concerning future directions
6. Questionable reasoning in experimental approach
7. Absence of acceptable scientific rationale
8. Unrealistic large amount of work
9. Lack of sufficient experimental detail
10. Uncritical approach.

Submission for publication

A paper is more likely to be published if it offers new information about an important topic that has been studied reliably. Editors have a responsibility to their readership and this is what they demand.

Advice on what to include and how a manuscript should be presented can be sought from experienced colleagues (even in other disciplines). The simplest and most important message is to follow a target journal's guidelines for authors exactly. Many authors do not do this and it annoys editors and reviewers to such an extent that it may jeopardize a fair assessment! Efforts at maximizing the presentation of the manuscript are more likely to be rewarded.

Manuscripts are usually set out with an Introduction, Methods, Results and Discussion. A clear, complete description of the study methodology (including statistical analyses[10]) is essential – a reader should be able to reproduce the study results. The discussion should follow a logical sequence: what were the study's main findings, how do they fit in with previous knowledge, what were the weaknesses (and strengths) of the study design, and what should now occur – a change in practice and/or further research?

The Consolidated Standards of Reporting Trials (**CONSORT**) statement has defined how and what should be reported in a **randomized controlled trial**.[37]* The essential features include identifying the study as a randomized trial, use of a structured abstract, definition of the study population, description of all aspects of the randomization process, clear study endpoints and methods of analyses, and discussion of potential biases.

* www.ama-assn.org.

References

1. Duncan PG, Cohen MM. The literature of anaesthesia: what are we learning? *Can J Anaesthesia* 1988; **3**:494–499.
2. Sackett DL, Haynes RB, Guyatt GH, Tugwell P. Deciding on the Best Therapy: A Basic Science for Clinical Medicine. Little Brown, Boston 1991: pp187–248.
3. Yusuf S, Collins R, Peto R. Why do we need some large, simple randomized trials? *Stat Med* 1984; **3**:409–420.
4. Myles PS. Why we need large randomised trials in anaesthesia [editorial]. *Br J Anaesth* 1999; **83**:833–834.
5. Rigg JRA, Jamrozik K, Myles PS. Evidence-based methods to improve anaesthesia and intensive care. *Curr Opinion Anaesthesiol* 1999; **12**:221–227.
6. Sniderman AD. Clinical trials, consensus conferences, and clinical practice. *Lancet* 1999; **354**:327–330.
7. Goodman NW. Making a mockery of research. *BMJ* 1991; **302**:242.
8. Goodman NW. Does research make better doctors? *Lancet* 1994; **343**:59.
9. Frieman JA, Chalmers TC, Smith H *et al.* The importance of beta, type II error and sample size in the design and interpretation of the randomized controlled trial. *N Engl J Med* 1978; **299**:690–694.
10. Gardner MJ, Machin D, Campbell MJ. Use of check lists in assessing the statistical content of medical studies. *BMJ* 1986; **292**:810–812.
11. Geller NL, Pocock SJ. Interim analyses in randomized clinical trials: ramifications and guidelines for practitioners. *Biometrics* 1987; **43**:213–223.
12. Pocock SJ. When to stop a clinical trial. *BMJ* 1992; **305**:235–240.
13. Brophy JM, Joseph L. Bayesian interim statistical analysis of randomised trials. *Lancet* 1997; **349**:1166–1169.
14. Department of Health. Ethics Committee Review of Multicentre Research. Department of Health, London 1997 (HSG[97]23).
15. Beales WB, Sebring HL, Crawford JT. Permissible medical experiments. From: The judgement of the Nuremberg Doctors Trial Tribunal. In: Trials of war criminals before the Nuremberg Military Tribunal, 1946–49 vol 2. US Government Printing Office, Washington, DC.
16. Shuster E. The Nuremberg Code: Hippocratic ethics and human rights. *Lancet* 1998; **351**:974–977.
17. World Medical Organisation. Declaration of Helsinki. *BMJ* 1996; **313**:1448–1449.
18. Gilbertson AA. Ethical review of research [editorial]. *Br J Anaesth* 1999; **92**:6–7.
19. Schafer A. The ethics of the randomised clinical trial. *N Engl J Med* 1982; **307**:719–724.
20. Ingelfinger FJ. Informed (but uneducated) consent [editorial]. *N Engl J Med* 1972; **287**:465–466.
21. Kopp VJ. Henry Knowles Beecher and the development of informed consent in anesthesia research. *Anesthesiology* 1999; **90**:1756–1765.
22. Madder H, Myles P, McRae R. Ethics review and clinical trials. *Lancet* 1998; **351**:1065.
23. Myles PS, Fletcher HE, Cairo S *et al.* Randomized trial of informed consent and recruitment for clinical trials in the immediate preoperative period. *Anesthesiology* 1999; **91**:969–978.
24. Freedman B. Equipoise and the ethics of clinical research. *N Eng J Med* 1987; **317**:141–145.
25. Hanna GB, Shimi S, Cuschieri A. A randomised study of influence of two-dimensional versus three-dimensional imaging on performance of laparoscopic cholecystectomy. *Lancet* 1998; **351**:248–251.
26. Cuschieri A. Ethics review and clinical trials (reply). *Lancet* 1998; **351**:1065.

27. Madder H. Existential autonomy: why patients should make their own choices. *J Ethics* 1997; **23**(4):221–225.
28. Zelen M. A new design for randomised clinical trials. *N Engl J Med* 1979; **300**:1242–1245.
29. Gore SM. The consumer principle of randomisation [letter]. *Lancet* 1994; **343**:58.
30. Truog RD. Randomized controlled trials: lessons from ECMO. *Clin Res* 1993; **40**:519–527.
31. Mingus IVIL, Levitan SA, Bradford CN, Eisenkraft JB. Surgical patient's attitudes regarding participation in clinical anesthesia research. *Anesth Analg* 1996; **82**:332–337.
32. Montgomery JE, Sneyd JR. Consent to clinical trials in anaesthesia. *Anaesthesia* 1998; **53**:227–230.
33. Tait AR, Voepel-Lewis T, Siewart M, Malviya S. Factors that influence parents' decisions to consent to their child's participation in clinical anesthesia research. *Anesth Analg* 1998; **86**:50–53.
34. Pearson KS. Emergency informed consent. *Anesthesiology* 1998; **89**:1047–1049.
35. Schwinn DA, DeLong ER, Shafer SL. Writing successful research proposals for medical science. *Anesthesiology* 1998; **88**:1660–1666.
36. Ogden TE, Goldberg IA. Research Proposals. A Guide to Success. 2nd ed. Raven Press, New York 1995: pp15–21.
37. Begg F, Cho M, Eastwood S *et al.* Improving the quality of reporting of randomized controlled trials. The CONSORT Statement. *JAMA* 1996; **276**:637–639.

13

Which statistical test to use: algorithms

The following algorithms are presented as a guide for new researchers, in order to assist them in choosing an appropriate statistical test. This is ultimately determined by the research question, which in turn determines the actual way in which the research should be designed and the type of data to collect.

In practice, there may be several other tests that could be employed to analyse data, with the final choice being left to the preference and experience of the statistician (or researcher). Many of these statistical tests are modifications of those presented here (and go under different names). Nevertheless, the choices offered here should satisfy most, if not all, of the beginner researcher's requirements. We strongly recommend the reader refer to the appropriate sections of this book in order to find more detail about each of the tests, their underlying assumptions, and how common mistakes can be avoided.

Each algorithm has three steps: (a) what type of research design is it, (b) what question is being asked, and (c) what type of data are being analysed. Further description of these issues can be found in Chapters 1 and 4.

The algorithms are given in Figures 13.1–13.4:

- to compare two or more independent groups – is there a difference? (Figure 13.1)
- to compare two or more paired (dependent) groups – is there a difference? (Figure 13.2)
- to describe the relationship between two variables – is there an association? (Figure 13.3)
- to describe the relationship between two measurement techniques – is there agreement? (Figure 13.4)

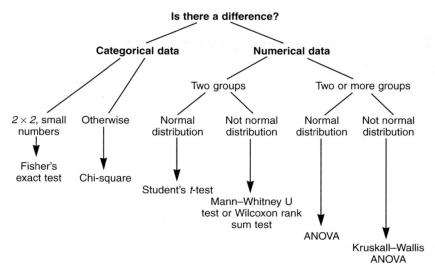

Figure 13.1 To compare two or more independent groups

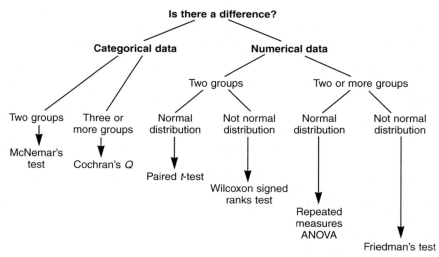

Figure 13.2 To compare two or more paired (dependent or matched) groups

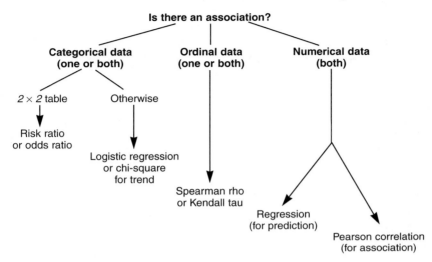

Figure 13.3 To describe the relationship between two variables

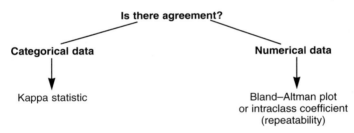

Figure 13.4 To describe the relationship between two measurement techniques

Index